Guidebooks for Counsel

Counsellors in the course of their prac
with particular difficulties, such as e)
addiction, or eating difficulties. These is
counselling and it may not be appropria   ... ull to a specialist
in one of these fields, if such exists locally. There may be literature available
but little guidance for the counsellor seeking it.

The Publications Committee of the British Association for Counselling are
publishing a series of booklets to help counsellors in this situation. Written by
specialist counsellors or therapists, they draw attention to issues which are
likely to arise for the client and for the counsellor and which may be missed
by the novice. They also provide a guide to the relevant literature. Being brief,
readable and to the point, it is hoped that counsellors will be able to consult
them even when time and money are short. In this way it is hoped that these
booklets will contribute to the raising of standards of counselling in general.

The Committee would like to thank not only those members who worked to
produce these booklets, but also Isobel Palmer and Sally Cook and the
consultant editors, myself, Gladeana McMahon and Stephen Palmer, whose
contribution was vital.

Julia Segal
Chair, Publications Committee of BAC from 1987 to 1993.

Dr Elphis Christopher MBBS DRCOG DCH IPM MFFP

Elphis Christopher is a medical doctor working in the field of family planning
and sexual medicine for almost 30 years. She has been a BAC member since
1977 and was Chair of PSMF Division 1980-1983.

She is a member of the Institute of Psychosexual Medicine and trained
recently as a Jungian therapist becoming an associ-
ate member in 1990 and a full member in 1994 of the
British Association of Psychotherapists.

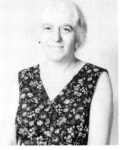

She is the author of Sexuality and Birth Control in
Community Work.

She has lectured widely and has made numerous
radio and TV appearances. After showing a condom
for the first time on British TV in 1975 in a secondary school sex education lesson she was accused of
being a 'crude and dangerous doctor'.

Counselling People with

Psycho-Sexual Problems

Dr. Elphis Christopher

British Association for Counselling
1 Regent Place • Rugby • Warwickshire CV21 2PJ
Office 01788 550899 • Information Line 01788 578328 • Fax 01788 562189

© BAC 1996   ISBN 0 946181 58 6

Published by: British Association for Counselling, company lim-
ited by guarantee 2175320 registered in England &
Wales, Registered Charity 298361

Printed by: Quorn Litho, Loughborough

Others in the Series

Counselling Adults who were Abused as Children by Peter Dale

Counselling People in Eating Distress by Carole Waskett

Counselling People with Infertility Problems by Sheila Naish

Working with Problem Drinkers by Mike Ward

British Association for Counselling

* Codes of Ethics & Practice for Counsellors, for Counselling Skills,
for Trainers in Counselling & Counselling Skills, for the Supervision
of Counsellors
* Counselling publications mail order service
* Quarterly journal with in-depth articles, news and views of members
* Individual, supervisor and trainer accreditation and counsellor train-
ing course recognition schemes
Join BAC now — the Voice of Counselling
Details of the above and much more besides:
BAC, 1 Regent Place, Rugby CV21 2PJ. Tel: 01788 550899

Contents

	Page
Introduction	1
Physiological Perspectives: The Sexual Response Cycle	5
Problems	
Types	7
Causes	9
Presentation	15
Treatment	18
Ethnicity	25
Issues for the Client	27
Issues for the Counsellor	28
Case Histories	32
Disabilities and Chronic Illness	
Physical	35
Learning Difficulties	39
Issues for the Client	39
Issues for the Counsellor	40
Parents of Children with Disabilities	41
Homosexuality	
In Men	43
Issues for the Client	44
Issues for the Counsellor	45
Lesbians	47
Issues for the Counsellor	48
Sexual Minorities	50
Sexual Offences	
Exhibitionism	58
Rape	58
Paedophilia	62
Useful Addresses	64
Recommended Book List	65

Foreword

Clients frequently bring anxiety about some aspect of sexuality to counsellors, and counsellors can sometimes feel out of their depth.

A glance at the contents page will indicate what a broad view is covered and readers should not miss out on the admirable introduction which defines psychosexual problems in simple terms and offers an overview of when and how these may occur and the effect they can have on individuals, families and on society as a whole.

Elphis Christopher gives us a wealth of information about many aspects of sexual difficulty ranging through intrapsychic conflicts, emotional aspects, relationships, physiological factors and the difficulties people with a disability may experience. She is supportive of both clients and counsellors and describes some of the issues that may arise for the client and those which may arise for counsellors where the focus is on particular difficulties. She outlines the various methods currently available for dealing with sexual problems and the sources of specialist help as well as providing a comprehensive reference list for those who want more detailed information on a specific topic.

Throughout the book we hear the author's sensitivity combined with a straightforward and down-to-earth approach which is encouraging to counsellors and, if they can develop the same qualities, will mean a great deal to clients who come to them in distress.

The constant references to sexual matters in the media these days make it very obvious that they are felt to be of great importance and also that they can evoke strong opinions and feelings. Dr. Christopher has been involved in a number of controversial issues over the years and in these she has been constant in speaking out on behalf of patients and clients, always giving priority to their needs. Twenty years ago I had the privilege of working with her in setting up the PSMF (now PSRF) Division of BAC and I am glad that she is sharing her wisdom and knowledge in this handbook. It will be of great use to counsellors who are not yet comfortable in helping those in sexual difficulty and a most useful update for those who are more experienced.

Mary Godden, BAC Accred
Fellow of BAC and Past Chair of BAC (1980-83)

Counselling People with Psycho Sexual Problems

Introduction

Psychosexual problems refer to sexual difficulties or dysfunctions which can affect physical function and are largely psychological or emotional in origin. While some sexual problems are due solely to physical causes these are not so common. The physical causes may be due to an inherited defect, disease, accident or the effect of ageing. However, even if there is a purely physical cause there is invariably an emotional reaction that can intensify the problem. Thus feelings affect function and vice versa.

The range of psychosexual problems is vast and varies in complexity and depth. Similarly treatment is variable both in type and length. Just one consultation may be sufficient or years of in-depth psychotherapy may be necessary. The problems may trouble the individual (intrapsychic); the couple (interpersonal); the family, as in sexual abuse or society as a whole with deviant antisocial sexual acts.

The people who often need the most help, for example, those committing antisocial sexual acts may not consult the counsellor until forced to by law. Others such as transvestites or those engaged in sadomasochistic or fetishistic acts may not see themselves as having any problem and only present for help when a partner is objecting to their behaviour. Sometimes it is the partner who seeks help.

The psychosexual problem may be a secondary phenomenon, a cover up as it were, for a much deeper psychological problem. Sadomasochistic and fetishistic acts come into this category where this behaviour is problematic and is compulsively repeated to relieve psychological tension and to prevent a psychotic breakdown. Such clients require years of therapy and can be difficult to treat.

There can be painful and complex issues to do with gender, sexual orientation, disability and disease. There may be enormous anxiety about what is 'normal' in terms of appearance, image, expectation, sexual functions, sexual behaviour and performance.

During the last 30 years western society's attitude towards sex has undergone a profound change. Sex is now a subject for open discussion, for newspaper and magazine articles, and for the media. Couples now expect to enjoy sex and are presenting themselves for treatment where there is a sexual problem. Perhaps the most significant change is to do with female sexuality. There is a general acceptance that women have a right to enjoy sex and have orgasms and to seek help if they experience difficulties.

Premarital sex for both sexes has become more common. With the advent of Gay Liberation in 1970, homosexuality began to be accepted as a valid expression of a person's sexuality rather than an illness to be treated. Increasing recognition has been given to the sexual needs of people with physical disabilities and learning difficulties.

Couples also hope to enjoy a sexual relationship free from the fear of unwanted pregnancy. Birth control methods are expected to be safe, convenient and effective. Increasingly some women are wanting not only easy access to abortion but the sole right to determine for themselves whether to have an abortion. The Abortion Act (passed in 1968) made the criteria for abortion less stringent. Since that time an increasing number of women are choosing to have an abortion rather than continue with an unwanted pregnancy.

Prior to this, Victorian attitudes to sex prevailed — albeit in somewhat diluted form: women were not supposed to be interested in or enjoy sex; premarital sex was frowned upon for girls, though tolerated for boys. These attitudes are still to be found especially among certain religious and cultural groups. These, broadly speaking, are the more patriarchal communities such as fundamentalist Christians and Jews, Greek and Turkish Cypriots and both Muslim and Hindu Asians.

The greater openness about sexuality has also revealed the extent of its dark side causing much shock to society – for example the sexual abuse of children and rape. During the 1980s the mood of optimism about sexuality was dampened. In 1981 the first cases of Acquired Immune Deficiency Syndrome (AIDS) were diagnosed. Initially it was often referred to by the media as 'the gay plague' since those affected at that time were thought to be mainly homosexual. AIDS is currently known to be spreading rapidly amongst heterosexuals, especially injecting drug users.

Infertility has become an increasingly noticeable problem with more women suffering from pelvic inflammatory disease resulting in blocked fallopian tubes. One in 6 couples has a fertility problem.

Although the incidence of syphilis and even gonorrhoea was beginning to fall, other sexually transmitted diseases have taken their place such as non-specific urethritis (NSU), chlamydia, herpes and viral warts. There has been an increase in the incidence of precancerous cell changes in the cervix (neck of the womb) in young women which, if untreated, may lead to cancer. There has also been a disenchantment with the most effective methods of contraception, especially the pill and intra-uterine device, despite the fact that the new lower dose oral contraceptive pills have been found to be much safer. Despite a free family planning service widely available through clinics and GPs the number of abortions has continued to rise (over 170,000 in 1993). All this has been seen by some as the inevitable consequences of the so-called revolution of the 60s and 70s. The prospect of couples having enjoyable sexual relationships free from the constraint of inhibition, fear, guilt and shame seems to have receded. The anxiety about AIDS has led to increased caution with the emphasis on safer sex (using the condom or being non-penetrative).

The majority of sexual difficulties (certainly those presenting to psychosexual clinics and counsellors) are to do with unsatisfactory heterosexual intercourse, though it is not possible to give accurate figures. Masters and Johnson estimated that one half of the marriages in the United States are threatened by sexual dysfunctions. An interesting study from the United States (Frank, Anderson and Ruberstein, 1978) analyzed the answers of 100 couples to a detailed self-report marital questionnaire. These couples were white, well-educated and 'happily married' (i.e. couples who thought their marriages were working). It was found that though 80% of the couples reported that their marital sexual relations were happy, 40% of men reported erection or ejaculation dysfunction and 63% of the women reported arousal or orgasmic dysfunction. It is unclear whether these difficulties were temporary or permanent. Whatever they were they did not seem to trouble the couple enough to seek help. It may be that when the relationship is working and sex reasonably satisfying, as reported by 86% of the women and 85% of the men in this study, people may be less inclined to seek any alteration. It perhaps needs to be stated that the perfect sexual performance (whatever that might be) is unlikely to be sustained on every sexual occasion. To expect it to be is to set the scene, paradoxically, for much sexual unhappiness. Three quarters of all couples who complain of sexual dysfunction also have marital difficulties and vice versa (Small, 1980). The most common sexual complaints presented at psychosexual clinics in the author's experience are problems with erection in men and loss of interest in sex in women.

Satisfactory solutions cannot be found for every problem but at least it should be possible for people to feel that problems can be aired and shared. Hopefully this should lead to greater understanding both of the self and one's relationships.

The range of psychosexual problems is vast. They can involve the individual or the couple. Certainly their effects can be far reaching – on the family or on Society itself. They can cause, often unnecessarily, a great deal of misery.

Not every counsellor can be an expert on sexuality and its problems. Nevertheless it is hoped that this booklet will go some way to enabling the counsellor to feel more knowledgeable and comfortable in listening to their client's sexual difficulties and distress and be more aware of what can be done to help. Hopefully too if out of their depth counsellors will be more aware of where to turn to for help both for themselves and more especially for their clients.

Physiological Perspectives: The Sexual Response Cycle

Masters and Johnson (a gynaecologist and psychologist respectively) working in St. Louis in the States, were the first workers to study the physiology – that is the bodily changes – of the human sexual response. They observed over 10,000 acts of sexual intercourse in 382 women aged 18-78 and 312 men aged 21-89 during the 1950s. This work was needed not only for the understanding of human sexuality but also to dispel myths and misinformation.

They discovered that the male and female sexual response was similar and they divided this into four phases.

1. Excitement (the penis through a reflex response becomes erect within 8 seconds and vagina enlarges and lubricates by means of sweating through its walls within 10-30 seconds).

2. Plateau (during which sexual excitement increases – the upper two thirds of the vagina balloons and the lower third decreases in width and depth forming the orgasmic platform, the uterus elevates into the pelvis, the penis increases its circumference and length).

3. Orgasmic (the most pleasurable of sexual sensations which results in ejaculation of semen in the male by means of rhythmic muscular contractions. In the woman, the muscles in the lower third of the vagina contract rhythmically. The force and intensity can vary).

4. Resolution: sexual organs return to the pre-excitement state.

Men require a refractory period of minutes in younger men to days in older men before they can be re-stimulated. Women are capable of being repeatedly stimulated to orgasm – the so-called multiple orgasms – without a refractory period.

Contrary to Freud's assumption, Masters and Johnson found that there were not two types of orgasm in the female – that is, clitoral and vaginal orgasm, but one only. They found that the vaginal musculature contracted rhythmically in orgasm whether the clitoris or vagina were stimulated and the changes seen were the same whether the women masturbated or had intercourse. What varied was the duration and the intensity of the orgasmic responses. However, Perry (1982) described two forms of orgasm. There is the orgasm that seems focused on the surface genitalia – the clitoris and the lower third of the vagina and a deeper one following penile thrusting which produces contractions of the uterus. This is perceived as more internal, deeper and fuller. These women describe orgasm which feels different from clitoral stimulation. There is probably a melding of the two kinds of orgasm. Some women only reach plateau phase and the sexual excitement dies away. These responses can obtain in the same women at different times. Up to 70% of women require concomitant direct clitoral stimulation during intercourse to achieve orgasm (Hite, 1978), 90% of women can experience orgasms with adequate stimulation but 10% have difficulty despite intense arousal. Only about 7% of women reach orgasm each time. Some women are quite happy without orgasms and do not find them necessary for sexual satisfaction. Orgasms can occur in both men and women during sleep and in some women during breast feeding.

When masturbating both sexes take about the same time to reach orgasm – 1-2 minutes in young men; 3-4 minutes in young women. However, during intercourse women generally take 12-13 minutes to complete the sex response cycle whereas men take a shorter time than this (about 4-10 minutes). Thus there needs to be an adjustment between the sexes to ensure that the woman is fully aroused. Masters and Johnson found that changes that occurred in the sexual cycle went on well into old age though at a slower rate. The man may not need to ejaculate on every sexual occasion. He can require more direct stimulation of the penis to obtain and sustain an erection. Women past the menopause may suffer from vaginal dryness unless they are receiving hormone replacement therapy. Vaginal lubrication during the excitement phase of the sexual response may take several minutes rather than a few seconds. Ignorance of these changes and anxiety about them can result in the man becoming impotent and sex being deliberately avoided by both sexes. The Americans have a short succinct phrase relating to sex and the elderly 'Use it or you lose it'; the longer sexual contact is avoided, the harder it will be to regain proper sexual functioning. Thus sexual difficulties in late, middle and old age can be prevented by timely advice and education. It may require a change in sexual attitudes as well as behaviour. For example, the man who has always 'taken the lead' may find it hard to let go and allow his partner to give him the increase in stimulation he needs. He may need counselling help in order not to feel that he is a failure or that this is somehow second best. He and his partner might gain from a new emphasis on the sensual aspects of lovemaking.

Types of Problems

Impotence or erectile failure 'Can't get it up'

Inability to obtain or sustain an erection. This can be primary where a man has never been able to penetrate the vagina (despite getting an erection when masturbating) or secondary where the man has previously functioned satisfactorily but then fails to obtain an erection. This is much more frequent than primary impotence. The experience of impotency is devastating for a man and is often described in terms of loss or death: 'I feel something has gone; a part of me is dead' are common descriptions. It has to be remembered that a man cannot consciously will an erection.

Between 10-20% of cases of impotence are caused by physical factors, for example, diabetes, rather than emotional and psychological ones. However, there will obviously be a psychological reaction to the problem which may well exacerbate it. Where the cause is physical the inability to obtain an erection will usually have a gradual onset. There will be no reflex morning erections with a full bladder or nocturnal erections in sleep. The man may still retain his sexual desire: 'I want to do it but nothing happens'.

Premature ejaculation 'Coming too soon'

This is a common problem particularly among young men. It usually improves with time, given that a man has a sympathetic partner. Kinsey (1948) reported that 75% of men ejaculate within 2 minutes of the initiation of intercourse. More recent studies show that the duration of intercourse for men is between 4 and 10 minutes (Morse, 1981). If premature ejaculation persists it may lead on to secondary impotence. It too is divided into primary and secondary where there has been good function previously. Men with premature ejaculation sometimes comfort themselves with the idea that they are highly sexed: 'She's only got to take her clothes off and I'm away'. Their partners, however, often lose interest in sex: 'It's all over before it's begun, so why bother?' is often the feeling experienced with underlying anger and disappointment. She indeed may be the partner who presents for help.

Ejaculatory incompetence

This is an uncommon sexual problem, often with deep psychological causes. A man can have an erection and maintain intercourse for a long time but not be able to ejaculate into the vagina. There is often ambivalence about possible parenthood in these men. The problem may well be first revealed at the infertility clinic when a woman states that she wants a child but has been unable to conceive.

Non-consummation

Full penetration by the penis has not taken place. Sometimes couples are uncertain whether penetration has been achieved and it is only when a vaginal examination has been attempted and the hymen is found intact that such a situation can be ascertained. Such women are often interested in sex, get sexually aroused and are orgasmic by manual stimulation. The non-consummation may have to do with fear of being vulnerable, of growing up or indeed of pregnancy. There may also be a wish – usually unconscious – to control the man by keeping him out despite behaving in a flirtatious and seductive way.

The partners of these women tend to be men who are not sexually confident: 'He's so kind he doesn't push it!' In some cases by not consummating the relationship the woman protects the man from knowing about his own impotence. Such couples tend to rely on mutual masturbation and tend to present when a child is wanted.

Painful intercourse

A woman often presents with complaints of pain whenever intercourse is attempted or occurs. She may complain about tightness, smallness or dryness. There can be a physical cause that needs appropriate treatment; alternatively, the discomfort may be due to the inability of the woman to become sexually aroused so that the normal sexual responses (enlargement of the vagina) do not take place.

Vaginismus

This refers to a clinical finding of spasms of the vaginal muscles. It can be so extreme as to prevent intercourse. It may arise from the fear of the pain of penetration. Where this persists the male partner may become impotent.

Orgasmic Dysfunction

Primary: the woman has never had an orgasm by any means.

Secondary: this can be further subdivided:

a)   the woman who has orgasm with intercourse but not on masturbation

b)   the woman who can achieve orgasm with masturbation and oral genital contact but not with sexual intercourse.

c)   the woman who occasionally gets orgasms, for example in special circumstances such as on holiday.

In a) the woman may feel that sexual intercourse alone is the only form of permissable sexual activity. In b) and c) there may be fears of 'letting go' and being overwhelmed with loss of control.

No interest in sex or general unresponsiveness

This can occur in both sexes and accompany the other conditions already mentioned and indeed may lead to them. It too can be divided into primary where there has never been much interest and secondary.

From studies so far available the commonest presenting problems are secondary impotence and premature ejaculation in the male and general unresponsiveness and lack of interest in the female.

Sexual problems can co-exist: for example, premature ejaculation in the man and secondary loss of interest or inability to get an orgasm in the woman.

Causes of Sexual Difficulties

Sexual difficulties are caused by a wide variety of factors. In some cases only one partner is affected, in others it is both. However where a problem presents in one partner, the other will eventually be affected.

Until recently it was thought that all sexual difficulties had their origins in faulty psychosexual development at a very early age due to forbidden, incestuous fantasies. These largely unconscious fantasies set up a conflict between the wish to enjoy sex and the fear of doing so. While unconscious intra-psychic factors may be of central importance in some people with sexual problems it has been appreciated that social and cultural factors also play their part. The overt and conscious ways of dealing with sex in the family can also result in sexual difficulties, not least the effects of sexual abuse and violence in the family. This has been given increasing recognition during the last 15 years. It can also be difficult to sort out whether the problem lies in the dynamics of this particular relationship or just in the sexual aspect of it. Thus there can be a chicken and egg situation with regard to what came first. Certainly disappointment or anger can be displaced into the sexual relationship especially where these are not openly confronted, one partner may, as a result withdraw sexually. The couple can then present as a 'sexual problem,' 'She's not interested any more'. The man finds he loses his erection before penetration or 'comes quickly'. It can be difficult to get to the repressed hostile hurt and angry feeling. Thus the conflict can be transferred to the bedroom with denial that anything is wrong with the relationship itself.

Ignorance

Many people are ignorant about their bodies, their sex organs and how they function. Ignorance is invariably accompanied by poor sexual technique. There may be false expectations of the sex act and the performance required of each partner. A common fallacy is that only men with large penises can give women orgasms. Thus if his partner does not get an orgasm the man may believe his penis is too small. The achievement of simultaneous orgasms without the use of hands is regarded by some as the epitome of the perfect sex act.

Fear

There may be a fear of intimacy and closeness, of sharing the good and the bad of oneself, of trusting and entrusting. There may be a fear of sex – fear of its power, fear of being overwhelmed or changed by it. There may be a fear of losing control. Joyful sex means abandonment, losing oneself, being playful and childlike. For some this is an experience which is too threatening. There is a fear of pain, of being damaged or of damaging a partner. Men may see the penis as a dangerous weapon and be afraid of their aggressive impulses. Influenced by feminism some men have tried to deny their aggressive feelings by becoming passive, believing that this is what women want.

A paradox then ensues: the woman is delighted that she has found a gentle, caring man but is dismayed that she does not find him sexually attractive. Such a man may express his anger by withdrawing or launching covert sadistic attacks. The man who fears the vagina (and the power of women) can ejaculate quickly in order to get out of such a potentially dangerous place. Both sexes may fear failure which then feeds on itself, one failure leading to another.

Fear can prevent sexual arousal (diverting blood that should go to the genital organs to the muscles) or switching off excitement once it has occurred. Masters and Johnson gave a special term ('performance anxiety') to the situation where a man who has previously failed to sustain an erection watches himself anxiously on each sexual encounter to see whether the problem will occur again. Unfortunately his so-called 'performance anxiety' ensures that erection will not take place. During foreplay the man may lose and then regain his erection. This can make a man so anxious once he thinks he has an erection he must use it instantly for fear of being unable to regain it.

Embarrassment, Shame and Disgust

These feelings are commonly associated with sex especially where it is believed that the 'good' person is a-sexual. Considerable guilt and shame may be experienced over sexual fantasies particularly those associated with masturbation. Disgust often manifests itself in an over-concern with personal hygiene or with a dislike of vaginal secretions and semen. Sex may be equated with 'mess', 'dirt' and 'excreta'. God can be seen as playing a trick on human beings by making the genital organ serve two functions (excretion and sex) in the case of the penis and being next to the organs of excretion in the case of the vagina – the temple of Venus next to the sewer.

Failure to Communicate and Unrealistic Expectations

Many couples with sexual difficulties have never discussed their own sexual feelings and desires. There may be a fear that doing so will be interpreted as criticism or rejection. Certain societal attitudes reinforce feelings, for example that men are expected to 'know' what to do. Consequently some men do feel threatened if their partners attempt to suggest what to do. Some women collude over this and 'fake orgasms'.

Unrealistic expectations may lead to disappointment which in time may cause resentment and hostility. Some women expect their partners to give them orgasms. Allied to this is a fantasy that somewhere there is a 'perfect' lover who will do all the right things. Some men feel they should be in charge and responsible for the woman's orgasm. Underlying this may be anxiety about potency or penis size. Some men are only potent if they are in charge and if the woman takes the sexual initiative he becomes impotent. What seems difficult for some couples to accept is that each partner is responsible for his or her own sexual feelings.

Collusive Patterns in Relationships

Certain sexual difficulties seem to go together and reflect the collusive adjustment which some couples make early on in their relationship. Only when one of the partners wishes to change (for whatever reason) will the difficulty of the other be unmasked. Thus the woman who is afraid of sex and her own sexuality may choose a sexually 'safe' man who makes few sexual demands. After marriage the woman may feel it is alright to be sexual whereupon she finds her partner is uninterested. She may then present with a complaint of losing her interest in sex. Men whose masculine image and potency on the belief that women are inferior tend to marry 'little girl' wives who are uncertain of their own sexuality. Sex may be satisfactory for a time but should the little girl grow up, the man may become impotent. Fear of powerful feelings, sexual excitement and anger cause some couples to exercise extreme control and denial of these feelings. They are often anxious to be seen as a 'nice couple' who never argue and so are under pressure to keep the relationship 'safe' and unexciting. Where there is an investment by both partners in being 'the same', sexual intercourse may be avoided because it demonstrates their difference.

Factors from the past influencing the present

Children are not born with sexual difficulties (unless these relate to a physical disability). The development of their sexuality and sexual confidence can be determined by many factors: the kind of family they grow up in, their relationships with their parents and siblings (and vice versa), their parents sexual relationship and their experience of adolescence.

Thus couples mentioned earlier who are afraid to show their feelings, including sexual ones, may have been reared in families where feelings were suppressed or denied. Alternatively, there may have been violent rows. This can lead to a fear of arguing (and being different) in case this leads to violence.

The capacity to form intimate and trusting relationships lies in a loving relationship with parents, especially the mother. For successful sexual relationships, the child needs to form a positive identification with the same sex parent. Where this fails to occur the person may despise his/her own sex and over value or envy the opposite sex. The sexuality of the child needs to be affirmed by both parents, especially by the opposite sex parent, without boundaries being crossed as in sexual abuse. Perceived or real failure in parenting can lead the child in later life to seek a parent substitute when sex can be a problem, as the partner is not seen as a lover. Unresolved feelings of anger, disappointment, envy or fear of the opposite sex parent may carry over to an adult sexual relationship. The man who is envious or fearful of women, for example, may disguise these feelings by idealising women. He may put his wife on a pedestal. She is then 'too pure' for him to sully with his dirty sexual desires. In frustrating her he punishes her whilst maintaining how much he worships and adores her. A failure to develop sexual confidence can occur where a sibling is thought to be more physically attractive and comparisons are constantly made either by the rival sibling or by the parents and other relatives.

Acceptance of the parents' sexual relationship as good and creative can influence how the child thinks about sex and his/her own sexuality. If the parents' sexual relationship is a poor one (for whatever reason e.g illness) a number of consequences may follow: The child may feel he/she has no right to enjoy sex later in life, the parent may turn to the child for comfort in an overt way (as in sexual abuse) or in covert ways binding the child emotionally. Thus a special relationship can be created e.g. daddy's girl, mother's boy thereby inhibiting or limiting the child's future sexual relationships. Separation – growing up and leaving home – is seen as a destructive and damaging act provoking much guilt. If the child has to care for an ill parent he/she may continue to seek to care for someone who represents a neglected self rather than be cared for realistically as an adult. The child may envy and resent the parent's relationship and feel they cannot compete and have a good sexual relationship of their own. Adolescence can be a difficult time with the young person trying to establish their sexual identity and explore whether they are sexually attractive. Rejections at this time can be particularly humiliating.

Although it may appear from the above that such attitudes are fixed, it should be noted that parents' attitudes towards their children are influenced by the children's own attitudes towards them. The significance of this for counsellors is that there can be a modification of such attitudes with counselling so that kinder feelings towards parents can give rise to kinder memories of parental behaviour. This can alter present behaviour towards the opposite sex.

Secondary Causes

These have to do with an altered life situation – stress of any kind, financial and domestic worries, fear of pregnancy, a difficult childbirth, birth of a handicapped child (see also chapter on Disabilities & Chronic Illness), guilt over an abortion, discovery of infertility, physical and mental health, fatigue, drugs used to treat illnesses, drug addiction, alcoholism, relationship or marriage break-up, an unfaithful partner, guilt over a secret affair, shame about past sexual behaviour, bereavement. The discovery of a sexually transmitted disease or an abnormal cervical smear can lead to a secondary sexual problem such as impotence or loss of interest in sex. Sexual boredom can occur possibly as a result of the predictability of always making love in the same way and in the same position. Sometimes if one partner wants the other to do something the other finds distasteful this can result in sexual difficulties. For example one partner may want oral sex which the other finds repugnant. Continued demand for it may eventually lead the other to switch off sexually. The partner whose sexual wishes are not met can end up feeling rejected and disgusted by their desires.

Couples who have enjoyed sex while living together can lose interest when married. It is 'legal' and expected. Sometimes such couples got married to try and save a failing relationship. Conflicts over children and the way they should be treated can cause relationship and sexual difficulties. Women may feel that once they become mothers they should not be lovers, especially if they believe their mothers did not enjoy sex.

Adults who were sexually abused as children

One of the dilemmas for the people involved in sexual abuse, where there is no violence or threat of it, is that their bodies may have involuntarily responded with pleasure. The shame and revulsion attached to this can also lead to later aversion to sex and self-disgust and the feeling that all sex is dirty. For such a person to allow herself to experience sexual desire will only confirm that she was really to blame for the abuse happening.

Presentation of sexual difficulties

Men and women differ in the frequency with which sexual problems are presented. More women than men used to complain of sexual difficulties at psychosexual clinics. Nowadays it is the author's impression that men are being increasingly referred. The sexes also differ in how they present the complaint and their perception of its cause: this has implications for treatment. Men tend to focus on the penis as if there were something wrong with the machinery which needs fixing. The connection between function and feeling is often denied (the 'below the waist' presentation). Women may have more diffuse complaints and seem to appreciate more readily that their general feelings of anger, sadness and disappointment can affect their sexual feelings (the 'above the waist' presentation).

Direct Complaint

Sexual problems can present overtly in a direct complaint that sex is painful or that there are difficulties in getting an erection. However the fact that people nowadays feel more able to state that they have sexual difficulties may divert the counsellor from looking at other problems which the individual (or couple) has but which are too painful to reveal.

Complaint about the partner

The man or woman can present with complaints about the partner's inadequacy or problem. These should not be accepted at face value. They may well conceal fears and anxieties about the self. For example, the man who complains that his partner's vagina is too large or that he does not get enough sensation is probably anxious that his penis is too small. Some people present themselves and their difficulties in a seemingly altruistic manner that can be very deceptive to the unwary. They usually present as being only there for the partner, saying they would not come for themselves as they are not really bothered. Deep resentment and disappointment can lie behind this seeming altruism. This will need to be confronted. The temptation is for the counsellor to join forces with the presenting partner against the absent one.

Medical and Gynaecological Problems

Emotional pain or conflict can be converted into physical pain. Thus sexual problems can present under the guises of tiredness, headaches and backaches, for which no physical cause can be found. Complaints by women of vaginal discharges and irregular prolonged periods can also indicate sexual difficulties. Sometimes a disability or chronic illness is used to hide a sexual problem arising from other causes.

Venerophobia (an obsessional fear of having a sexually transmitted disease) or repeated induced abortions can cover up a sexual problem linked to shame and guilt for having sexual desires and sexual relationships.

After hysterectomy or sterilisation both men and women may lose interest in sex. They may fail to mourn the loss of their ability to produce children and may feel they are no longer a 'real woman' or a 'real man'.

Contraceptive Problems

There can be conflict over the method used, over which partner uses a method, or whether contraception is used. Sometimes these conflicts are to do with envy and resentment of the partner's sexual needs and a wish to control or limit them by not using contraception. Where sex is regarded solely for procreation and not for pleasure there can be difficulty in choosing and/or persevering with a method. Sometimes individuals or couples can only allow themselves to become sexually excited when there is a risk of pregnancy. This can lead to a 'contraceptive roulette'. Methods can be scapegoated for causing a loss of interest in sex. Ambivalence towards contraception can occur when one partner secretly wants a pregnancy.

Infertility Problems

Infertility can be caused by and be the cause of sexual difficulties. Non-consummation, impotence, ejaculatory incompetence can all present as an infertility problem. The knowledge that the couple or one of the partners is infertile can lead to sexual difficulties, such as a loss of interest in sex. It is estimated that about one in six couples are infertile in Britain (around 2 million people). Although women have been blamed in the past for infertility – the barren woman of the Bible – present knowledge shows that 30-35% of cases are due to male problems, 30-35% to female, with 30% due to a combination of the two. A contributory factor is that many women, especially professional women are delaying their first pregnancy until their mid to late 30s. Women are most fertile in their 20s, their fertility declining thereafter. It has been estimated that about 50-60% of all infertility can be treated if the couple has access to expert medical care. That leaves a large number of people who will have to cope with the knowledge that they are infertile. Some manage to get on with their lives, others go through a long mourning process for which they need help and support. Counselling is needed before, during and after investigations and treatment (see Sheila Naish *Counselling People with Infertility Problems* BAC Booklet, 1994). Sexual relationships can be affected at any stage and the relationship itself may not survive.

Before the investigations couples may be concerned about the psychological and emotional implications of treatment as well as the cost, length and discomfort. Ambivalence about having children may not be admitted. However, it may manifest itself by infrequent sex or expressed in anxieties about the cost of treatment.

During investigations and treatment, the stress involved when couples live in 'the cycle of hope and despair' can actually result in the semen and cervical mucus becoming poor in quality and menstrual cycle altering. Although the tests can be reassuring in the sense that something is being done, they can have a de-humanising effect. Sex itself can become a mechanical, self-conscious, joyless act.

When the results show something definitely wrong in one partner while the other is normal, a great strain can be put on the relationship. The partner with the abnormality can feel a 'freak', less of a man or woman and sexually undesirable. Treatment such as artificial insemination using donor sperm (AID) or in vitro fertilisation may add to feelings of inadequacy leading to impotence or other problems. Counselling couples with infertility problems is especially poignant and painful. The couples are usually healthy people enjoying their lives. The experience of infertility can have devastating effects changing a person's self image and the personal and sexual relationship. For some there will be the longed for baby making things 'normal'. For others who fail to have a child life will not be the same again, so many losses will have to be mourned, sex may cease to be enjoyable and the relationship may end. The counsellor's task will be a difficult one trying to help the couple restore some faith in themselves and their capacity to enjoy their lives again including their sexual lives.

Problems Associated with Pregnancy and Childbirth

Sexual problems such as a loss of interest in sex can occur after an abortion, miscarriage or stillbirth, especially where the woman has been prevented from discussing her feelings about what has happened. Sexual problems frequently present after a new birth, especially the first. Some women believe the task of having sex is now accomplished, lose interest in it and take on a 'Madonna' image, i.e. mothers cannot be lovers. Much of this feeling is a carry-over from childhood feelings that their own mothers were asexual beings. In new mothers there is an emotional absorption with the baby which can make the husband/ partner feel excluded. There is the physical reality of tiredness, broken nights and the emotional demands of a baby that may well make the woman uninterested in sex. If the husband is immature and needs his wife as a mother also, he may begin to make impossible demands on her, sexually and otherwise, which lead to resentment. Extramarital affairs can take place at this time. A painful delivery can also lead to a loss of interest in sex in the woman and a fear on the part of the man about damaging his partner and/or damaging his penis. After childbirth some women feel the vagina no longer belongs to them – it has been 'medicalised'. If the woman feels unsupported by her partner she can lose sexual interest.

Treatment

It used to be thought that most sexual difficulties resulted from unresolved oedipal conflicts originating in childhood and hence could only be helped by prolonged analysis. The work of doctors belonging to the Institute of Psychosexual Medicine and the use of Masters and Johnson sex therapy techniques by counsellors and psychologists have shown that many sexual problems can be treated more quickly and less expensively. Although psychoanalysis is not a form of therapy available to most people, the insights derived from the work of psychoanalysts are nevertheless used by many counsellors and sex therapists. For those who do manage to obtain analysis general improvement in relationships and a considerable enhancement of sexual life, in particular, is a common experience. Psychodynamic psychotherapy may also improve relationships by working with the individual's unconscious conflicts. Long term work may be required to bring about changes in some aspects of sexuality, others may change more easily. Where a relationship, including sexual relationship, has been good in the past and some event had changed it for the worse there would be a better hope of helping a couple to regain their previous relationship or improve it.

The dilemma facing the client and the counsellor is knowing which is the best treatment for a particular problem. The client (and counsellor) may see a sexual difficulty as a medical problem, rather than an emotional or physical one. Help may then be sought from the general practitioner in the first instance. The counsellor may feel intimidated by the presentation of a sexual problem and wish to transfer the client to a specialist agency thereby avoiding exploration of the problem and the possible help s/he can give. This will be examined later under issues for the counsellor.

The brief psychotherapy/psychosomatic approach as practised by those doctors trained by the Institute of Psychosexual Medicine and the sex therapy techniques of Masters and Johnson are described below both to inform and enable the counsellor to make an appropriate referral. As a general rule sex therapy may be most useful for couples where both partners present for help and where the relationship is basically a good one. If there are problems with the relationship (other than the sexual aspect) the appropriate referral may be to a Relate counsellor. If an individual seeks help for a sexual problem, referral to a psychosexual doctor may be indicated, especially if a physical examination is also required.

Brief Psychotherapy – the Psychosomatic or Balint-Main Approach

Sexual problems were (and are) often presented at a family planning clinic. They were consciously stated or unconsciously revealed through feelings of ambivalence over contraception and fear of the vaginal examination. Doctors working at these clinics were conscious of their lack of expertise in this area.

In the late 1950s a group of family planning doctors approached Michael Balint (then working as an analyst at the Tavistock Clinic) with a view to devising a training scheme along the lines Balint was using to train general practitioners. Balint helped to start, and Dr. Tom Main carried on the so-called seminar training technique in which a group of about 8 members meet fortnightly under the leadership of a trained doctor over the course of 1-2 years. Cases are presented and the focus is on the doctor-patient relationship. The aim is to try to understand what the patient is really saying and meaning and how emotional factors (not always fully conscious) are preventing the patient enjoying sex. The doctor tries to understand the communication by thinking about what   s/he feels with this particular patient and to reflect this back to the patient. For example, the person who expects the doctor to do all the work without revealing very much may well be doing this to the partner. The doctor, rather than ignoring this and his own angry feelings about being 'used' can comment on it to the patient and suggest that perhaps this is what the patient is doing to the partner. The patient may reveal that there are a lot of angry, resentful feelings towards the partner which have been bottled up. The doctor can then explore with the patient why it is so hard to express these feelings. This can be linked to something in the past such as a parent or sibling who bullied the patient. Thus use is made of the 'here and now' of the situation and the current doctor-patient relationship can link with the 'there and then' in the past, thus providing the patient with insight into why s/he is behaving in a particular way. Precisely who is complaining and who is the real 'patient' has to be determined.

The genital examination can be used by the psychosexual doctor to diagnose and treat sexual problems (the psychosomatic approach). A woman might not consciously admit to a sexual problem but the finding of tight vaginal muscles (vaginismus) by the doctor, when explained to the woman allows her to talk about it. The woman is then encouraged to examine her vagina with her fingers and to disclose her fantasies about her vagina while doing so. It is understandable that women should have fantasies about their bodies since their sex organs (unlike a man's) are hidden. Girls are often admonished by their mothers if they do try to explore themselves. They may believe that the vagina is too small (this can also refer to themselves – they are not grown up enough for sex). Examination can offer reassurance and the doctor can at the same time give permission to the woman to own her vagina and accept it as a good part of herself.

Treatment is focused on the presenting partner, oedipal conflicts are not dealt with in depth and the aim is to treat in 5-10 sessions. The other partner is not requested to attend but if s/he does then the work will continue with the partner as well as with the couple if they attend together. Around 1600 doctors (including GPs and hospital doctors) have done the basic training. The doctors so trained may use their expertise in general practice or community clinic. The Institute of

Psychosexual Medicine (IPM) was formed in 1975 taking over the training function from the Family Planning Association. There is now a Diploma in Psychosexual Medicine. It has a membership of around 400 doctors. There are about 60-70 psychosexual clinics in Britain. The majority are run by the NHS and are free. About 4-6 couples are seen in a session.

Masters and Johnson Behaviourist Techniques: Sex Therapy

Masters and Johnson followed up their research into the physiology of the sexual response by looking at and devising treatments for heterosexual difficulties. Although treatment is often considered 'behaviourist'. Masters and Johnson have also stated they gave 'psychotherapy to the relationship', that is, helping the couple deal with the conflict and destructive feelings which threaten the relationship.

This way of working requires that:

a)   An extensive sexual history is taken, ascertaining the attitudes, feelings and values of the couple regarding sex, their previous sexual experiences, and also clearing up misinformation. The relationship and interaction of the couple is assessed.

Male and female co-therapists are considered essential by Masters and Johnson (though not by later workers e.g. Helen Singer Kaplan, Bancroft) in order to have same gender advocate for each partner. Round-table discussions are held as well as separate interviews between each partner and one of the therapists. A medical history and examination are also undertaken (one of the therapists was a doctor).

b)   The couple are forbidden to have intercourse but are told to concentrate on 'pleasuring' each other by means of touching and stroking (not genitals) – the sensate focus. This has two purposes:

    i. It takes the emphasis off achievement and lessens the anxiety of 'spectatoring', i.e. the person observing himself, and

    ii. It helps the couple become aware of their own and their partner's bodily sensations.

c)   Once the sensation focusing is successful then special techniques are taught for each difficulty. Daily discussions are held with the therapist to discuss the couple's progress and prescribe the next sequence of treatment. Originally, Masters and Johnson advised a three-week residential course for treatment. Other workers such as Helen Singer Kaplan see couples weekly.

It is important to stress that Masters and Johnson selected their patients carefully. They insisted on referral by an authority. Couples were told about the Masters and Johnson approach and strong motivation was expected. Thus couples were only accepted where both partners were really interested in reversing their dysfunction and the relationship was stable. Their results were extraordinarily good. In the Masters and Johnson study 510 couples were treated and followed up for 5 years. Masters and Johnson used an unusual method of reporting outcome – by giving the failure rate rather than the success rate. Thus there was a 2% failure rate for premature ejaculation; a 26% failure rate for secondary impotence; and a 16% failure rate for dysfunction in women. The criteria used for assessing failure varied for each type of dysfunction. For example, erectile impotence failure was adjudged if erection sufficient for intercourse was not maintained in at least 75% of opportunities. Women with orgasmic dysfunction were failure if they 'did not reach orgasm in a consistent fashion during sexual opportunities . . .' 50% being a general guide. Small, I.F. 1980.

Sufficient time has now elapsed to evaluate the success rates of other workers both in the United States and in Britain using modified Masters and Johnson techniques, i.e. seeing couples weekly rather than daily, using one therapist rather than two. No other workers have matched the success of Masters and Johnson. Wright (1977) and Cole (1985) and Hawton (1995) have reviewed several independent studies. Crown (1983) has commented that sex therapy as practised at the moment seems to lead to improvement in around two thirds of patients presenting with sexual problems to outpatient clinics known to have a special interest in their treatment. It has proved difficult to follow up couples who have been treated and in those who have been contacted there has been quite a high relapse rate. Bancroft (1989) has explored the difficulties inherent in evaluating the outcome of sex therapy. It is easier, for example, to assess whether vaginismus has been 'cured' by sex therapy techniques compared to low sexual desire.

Perhaps of greater interest to the counsellor is the study of Crowe et al. (1981) comparing a modified Masters and Johnson approach using one or two therapists with one focusing on marital problems, emphasising contracts and improving communication. This study showed improvement in all techniques and no significant difference between them.

Helen Singer Kaplan (herself an analyst) has favoured a format that 'provides the opportunity for intensive conjoint and individual psychotherapy with the systematic prescription of sexual experience.' Her therapists are psychotherapeutically trained. The emphasis is on attempting to deal with the sexual problem at a superficial level then to work with resistances and defence in the person and the relationship as these block behavioural treatment.

Present position in Britain regarding Masters and Johnson techniques

Modified Masters and Johnson techniques are being used by:

a) Doctors who have been trained through the Institute of Psychosexual Medicine. However the use of Masters and Johnson is not their main treatment approach.

b) Several psychiatric and psychological departments in NHS hospitals.

c) Some Relate (marriage guidance) counsellors who have been trained in Masters and Johnson techniques since 1976 and run 'Marital Sexual Therapy Clinics' (MST). There are now around 60 such clinics. A small fee may be charged.

d) Sex therapists in private practice.

To sum up: Whilst it is true that many sexual difficulties are of a superficial nature needing only re-education others are more complex and include psychological conflicts in one or both partners together with relationship and marital difficulties. These may need to be treated either before or in conjunction with the sexual problem.

Conjoint therapy: This means more than one therapist, often one male and one female, so that each can act as advocate for the client of their own gender. The relationship between them can also be used as a model by the couple.

Psychosexual doctors and Relate counsellors usually work singly – co-therapists are not essential. However it is essential that the psychosexual worker understands the sexual reactions and needs of both genders.

Other Approaches

Films, books and sex aids (such as vibrators)

These have been used by some workers in conjunction with Masters and Johnson techniques in order to free couples from their inhibitions and to give them permission to explore their own sexual fantasies and what excites them.

Couples Groups

Couples with sexual difficulties are brought together to discuss and share their problems.

Medical Treatments

These are now available for impotence caused by physical factors such as diabetes or multiple sclerosis.

1) Papaverine injection given directly into the penis – the man is taught to do this himself. This drug acts on the blood vessels in the penis dilating them. This treatment is available from certain Urology Outpatient Departments. These injections produce a good response in men who have nerve damage but not those who have severe vascular disease. A more recently discovered drug, caverject (a prostaglandin) is said to be more beneficial.

2) Non-invasive techniques such as Erec Aid. A vacuum is created around the penis allowing it to swell and then a rubber band is placed on the base of the penis to maintain the erection for up to half an hour when the rubber band has to be released. The devices are not available on the NHS. They can be obtained through special medical suppliers and cost around £250. (They can be obtained from Osbon Medical, 29 Pattison Road, NW2 2HL)

3) Penile Prosthesis. Surgical implants of silicon rods into the penis. Again these are available in certain Urology Departments.

4) Vascular surgery to the penis where there is arterial damage or venous leak.

It is unfortunate that counselling for the man and his partner is not always available with the medical treatments. Follow up studies of these methods of treatment have shown that the partner or wife of the man expressed less satisfaction with them when she was interviewed alone.

Ethnicity and Sexual Problems

Although it may appear that sexual problems are only prevalent in Western Society with its Judaeo-Christian tradition, they are in fact found in every ethnic group. Anxiety about sex and sexual performance seems universal. Whether and how the problems present and what is expected from treatment may differ. Attitudes towards sexuality and adherence to cultural norms depend heavily on educational level and religious conformity – those who are less well-educated and more conformist are more likely to maintain cultural norms. The level of education and degree of sophistication can also determine whether a person complains of a sexual problem directly, who presents it and what expectations there are for treatment.

Many individuals may well be at a transitional stage between their culture of origin and that of Britain. This can lead to inter-generational conflict between those (usually the old) who wish to preserve their culture and those (usually the young) who wish to abandon it either wholesale or partially. This is particularly relevant to those practices relating to sex, marriage and the family.

Patriarchal – Asian, Cypriot

In these cultures sex education is almost totally lacking except that relating to personal hygiene and the need for modesty especially in girls. Among Moslems the genital organs are accorded special respect and must only be touched with the left hand. Masturbation is frowned upon and homosexuality is regarded as abnormal. Virginity is expected of girls before marriage. Marriages are arranged and can be more in the nature of a business transaction than a love match. Sex is regarded as a duty which must result in children, particularly sons. For the man to admit he has a sexual problem means extreme loss of face and the woman can be blamed for the problem. Contrary to what might be expected in a male-dominated society, sexual problems are common among men. This can be caused by the economic expectations put on a man to provide for his extended family – an expectation which might be impossible to fulfil. There is great anxiety about confidentiality and need to keep the families of both husband and wife in ignorance. In-law trouble appears to be quite common: the wife feels resentful both of her mother-in-law's interference and her close relationship with her son.

She (the wife) may not feel able to complain so she withdraws sexually or presents with a variety of symptoms. Couples are likely to have difficulty in discussing their feelings since the family is considered all important so less attention is paid to the needs or desires of individuals. Women rarely present with sexual difficulties directly: it is far more probable that a difficulty will be presented indirectly, as a problem connected with anxiety about conceiving. Language difficulties often present an additional hurdle.

Afro-Caribbean

Sexual activity and sexual pleasure for both sexes seems more acceptable in these cultures. The double standard of morality is not so much in evidence. Both masturbation and homosexuality are regarded as abnormal. Sex is likely to be discussed openly between couples. Women tend to be more openly critical of their partners: 'He's no good to me' indicates that the male partner is impotent. Men can be anxious lest they do not please their women sexually. Once a sexual problem does occur it can be difficult for the individual to accept that there is no physical cause since sex is seen as a natural function.

Issues for the Client

- There may be embarrassment and shame in talking about sex and sexual feelings. Is this the 'right' place? Is the counsellor the 'right' person?

- The client may question whether the counsellor can be trusted with such intimate matters. Is it safe? Thus it may only be after the client has been seeing the counsellor for some time that the sexual difficulty can be mentioned.

- There may be uncertainty/awkwardness about language.

- The client may be anxious about age/sex of the counsellor and disparity with client's age. For example an older man might feel intimidated talking about his erectile problems with a vigorous-looking young man whom he may fantasise will be contemptuous of him.

- The client may fear exposing ignorance or sexual abnormality or 'abnormal' sexual fantasies and desires.

- The client may be concerned about confidentiality especially with regard to the partner, e.g. a married man experiencing difficulty with his wife and finding he is attracted to other men.

- Differences between client and counsellor as regards ethnic group, health status, marital status or sexual orientation may concern the client. A disabled or minority group counsellor may be seen as 'second best': a dominant group counsellor may be seen as demanding deference and being unable to empathise.

Issues for the Counsellor

*   The counsellor needs to develop a relaxed attitude when talking about sexual matters.

*   The counsellor needs to be comfortable with sexual language and be aware of the euphemisms for genital organs and sexual function. This is not to say that the counsellor needs to use four-letter words when talking about sex but they must convey that they do understand what the client means – if they do not they should be able to check it out with the client.

*   The counsellor needs to be informed about sexual issues and sources of help.

*   The counsellor needs to be non-judgmental and guard against imposing their own ideas about what is sexually or culturally normal.

*   The counsellor needs to be aware that a sexual problem may be hidden by other problems that the client brings. For example, a male client may be depressed and anxious about being made redundant. He may secretly fear what this will do to his marriage; that he feels less of a man but be too embarrassed to talk about it. The counsellor could open up the topic by saying something like 'I wonder what you feel this will do to your relationship with your wife and both your sexual needs.'

*   The counsellor needs to be aware that the opposite is also true. The presentation of a sexual problem may hide another problem that the client finds more difficult to discuss. For example, a woman complained of losing interest in sex and wondered whether it was 'because of the pill'. It took some time before it emerged that she was grieving for a pregnancy which she had terminated. Once she had mourned the loss of the pregnancy she regained her interest in sex.

It is worth the counsellor asking themselves, and the client, why the problem has become important now, especially where it has persisted for some time. Where the sexual problem is of recent origin it is worth asking what else has changed in the client's life. The solution to the sexual difficulty may lie in the answer. For example, a woman may not have shown any interest in sex and not let it bother her for years. Suddenly she seeks help. What is going on? It could be that she has discovered that her husband has been having an affair and she wants to save her marriage.

- The sexual problem must not be regarded as something separate from the whole person. Thus when a man complains he cannot get an erection the counsellor must remember that the man himself feels impotent not just his penis.

- The counsellor needs to guard against sending for the partner especially when the client seems to be putting all the blame on him/her. The counsellor needs to 'stay with' the client and try to understand what is going on.

- The counsellor needs to be aware of getting trapped in to stereotypical views with a client such as 'All men are bastards, rapists, sexual abusers' or 'All women are 'castrating bitches, wanting to swallow you up.'

- The counsellor needs to remember that some sexual difficulties can be due to ignorance – any misunderstanding or misinformation can be corrected but obviously they need to be discovered first.

- The counsellor can be a 'good' parent enabling clients to express their feelings and admit their sexual interests and desires.

- The counsellor if he/she works alone may need to hold on to their own sexual identity while being aware of their contrasexual aspects. This can better facilitate empathy with their clients.

- The counsellor can enable better sex communication between partners.

- The use of Masters and Johnson techniques by the counsellor untrained in them is controversial. Counsellors risk getting out of their depth and also disillusioning the couple about the efficacy of sex therapy. The biggest pitfall is the quality of the couple's relationship. Masters and Johnson techniques only work when there is a good relationship without any underlying hostility or resentment that could sabotage treatment. One way of testing the presence of those feelings is to suggest sensate focusing; that is, for the couple to spend time each evening, say 20 minutes for about 1-2 weeks, caressing and stroking each other in turn in a non-demanding way, i.e. without the expectation of sexual intercourse. Failure to do this usually exposes the underlying hostility which can then be confronted.

- Seduction Issue: (Rutter, 1990) There is an understandable anxiety about seduction whenever sexual problems are raised. Will the counsellor be accused by the client's partner of attempting to seduce the client? The counsellor may find themselves attracted to the client. These feelings will be inevitable from time to time. The counsellors may use their feelings to affirm the sexual attractiveness of the client who feels sexually unattractive. However, the counsellor needs to make it clear by manner and/or words where the boundaries lie and that they will not be crossed. This is similar to the good parent who affirms their teenage child's sexual attractiveness but does not attempt to have a sexual relationship.

- The client may sexualize the interview to divert the counsellor from looking at his sexual fears and inadequacies or from other painful areas. The counsellor rather than ignoring what is happening can say something like 'You seem to find it easier to be sexual with me rather than work with me as a counsellor'.

- Referral: If the counsellor is getting out of their depth they must acknowledge it to themselves and the client and be prepared to refer the client elsewhere. This is often easier said than done, not least because there may be no local specialist agency.

If an attachment has been formed, referral can be difficult as the client could interpret this as rejection. This will need to be addressed before referral is made. The counsellor may feel understandable envy for the sex therapist or psychosexual doctor who is 'the expert'. The successful outcome of treatment may hinge on how a referral is made and whether it is appropriate. Sometimes it can be done to get rid of the difficult or unpleasant client – the counsellor comforting themselves that they are 'leaving no stone unturned', but in reality dumping the client.

Some guidelines on referral

The counsellor should:

1. Get to know the agency/personnel who are offering treatment.
2. Find out what kind of treatment is offered.
3. Find out whether therapy is given by a single therapist or co-therapists.
4. Find out whether the individual is treated or whether the couple have to attend.

5.   Find out the possible length of treatment and commitment required of the client.

6.   Find out how to refer (self-referral, direct referral or through the GP).

Sometimes it may be appropriate for the counsellor to continue seeing the client. This will need to be clarified with the therapist to avoid competition and/or manipulation by the client.

Case Histories

Guilt about premarital sex

Mr and Mrs B were referred by their GP to a psychosexual doctor. The complaint was painful intercourse. Mrs B complained of headaches and stomach aches and was awaiting hospital investigation for these. She was well-dressed in a rather severe way with gloves, hat and umbrella. Mr B, who was more casually dressed, was angry and resentful. It later emerged that he had developed premature ejaculation in order to get intercourse over with quickly after Mrs B's complaints of pain. Exploration of guilt surrounding their premarital sexual activities (they were both strict Catholics and had had a 'lovely white wedding') together with vaginal examination and self-examination with permission given to be sexual by a parent figure resulted in a cure after three sessions. The hospital appointment was cancelled and Mr B's premature ejaculation also ceased.

Vaginismus

Miss C attended a clinic where vaginismus was discovered on routine examination. She refused to examine herself. She was seen regularly over the course of a year. When she was a child her parents had fought over money and sex (her mother wanted the money and her father the sex). Mother kept Miss C in bed with her and she witnessed repeated scenes of father coming to mother and wanting sex which mother refused 'because of Miss C.' Miss C grew up believing that she had denied mother a sex life and she must therefore punish herself by denying herself, too. Father's visits had also made her excited but afraid, so while she could allow herself to get excited (she had had many boyfriends) she could not let them in. When eventually she understood and accepted that if mother and father had really wanted sex she could not have stopped them, it enabled her to give herself permission to have sex herself.

Premature ejaculation

Mr D attended a clinic, sad and depressed. he 'came too quickly' and his wife was getting fed up. This had not bothered them in the past but recently there had been a lot more worries and he found it increasingly difficult to cope. It emerged that he had set up his own business and was finding it difficult to confront his employees when they failed to do a job properly. He usually ended up doing the job himself and came home exhausted. Sex had become an 'on-off' experience. His wife also grumbled that he did not share his problems with her any more. Several sessions were spent exploring these *difficulties with him alone. He began to regain his confidence and managed to 'stand up to' his bank manager. He also confided more in his wife who was able to comfort him. Sex improved as they gave more time to each other.*

Secondary impotence

Mr E was a man in his 60s. His general practitioner's letter stated that he was a widower of several years and that he now had a new partner with whom he hoped to settle down but was unable 'to perform'. Although Mr E seemed to talk quite freely about his sexual difficulties the psychosexual doctor found herself sad and despondent. It was as if Mr E had brought something in with him but was trying to ignore it. The doctor decided to confront this by saying that there seemed to be a feeling of sadness around as if Mr E were not really free. At this time Mr E began to cry softly and talk about his 'beloved wife'. At the end of this session he said he was surprised at himself. He thought he had 'got over' the death of his wife but recalled that he had actually never had time to cry; so much had had to be done to keep going, the business they ran together and look after their teenage children. It was only after considerable 'mourning work' had been done that Mr E did feel 'free' to consummate his new relationship.

References

1. Kinsey, AC, Pomeroy, WB & Martin CE (1948) *Sexual Behaviour in the Human Male*. Philadelphia: WB Saunders.
   Kinsey, AC, Pomeroy, WB & Martin, CE (1953) *Sexual Behaviour in the Human Female*. Philadelphia: WB Saunders.
2. Cole, M & Dryden, W (eds) (1988) *Sex Therapy in Britain*. Open University Press.
3. Wellings, K et al. *Sexual Behaviour in Britain* (1994) Penguin
4. Masters, WH & Johnson, VE (1966) *Human Sexual Response*. Boston MA: Little Brown & Co.
5. Perry, JD & Whipple, B (1982) *Multiple Components of the Female Orgasm*. Circumvaginal Musculature & Sexual Function.
   Ed. Graber, D. Karger: Omaha.
6. Hite, S. (1976) *The Hite Report*. Macmillan Publishing Co.
7. Frank, E, Anderson, C & Ruberstein, D (1978). *Frequency of Sexual Dysfunction in 'Normal' Couples*. The New England Journal of Medicine, 229(3), 111-115.
8. Small, I.F. & Small, J.G. (1980) *Psychosexual Dysfunction*. In Comprehensive Textbook of Psychiatry III Ed. Kaplan, HI, Freidman, AM & Sadock,BJ. Williams & Wilkins: Baltimore.
9. Morse, WI & Morse, JM (1981) *Coital Premature Ejaculation with Masturbatory Ejaculation Incompetence*. Journal of Sex Education and Therapy, Vol. 7 No. 1, pp. 3-6

10. Skrine, RL (ed) (1989) *Introduction to Psychosexual Medicine.* Montana Press.
11. Tunnadine, LPD. (1983). *The Making of Love.* CAPE.
12. Kaplan, HS (1974) *The New Sex Therapy.* New York: Brunner Mazel. London: Balliere Tindail.
13. Bancroft, J. (1989) *Human Sexuality and its Problems.* 2nd Edition. Chuchill Livingstone.
14. Wright, J, Perrault, R & Mathieu, M (1977) *The Treatment of Sexual Dysfunction.* Archives of General Psychiatry, 34.
15. Cole, M. *Ch.2* (1988) in *Sex Therapy in Britain* Eds. Cole, M & Dryden, W. Open University Press.
16. Hawton, K. (1995) *Treatment of Sexual Dysfunctions by Sex*
Therapy and other approaches. British Journal of Psychiatry. 167, 307-314
17. Crown, S & d'Ardenne, P (1982) *Controversies, Methods and Results in Sex Therapy.* British Journal of Psychiatry, 140, 70-77.
18. Crow, MJ, Gillan, P & Golumbok, S (1981). *Form & content in the Conjoint Treatment of Sexual Dysfunctions: A Controlled Study.* Behaviour Research & Therapy, Vol. 19,pp.47 & 54.
19. Rutter,P. (1990) *Sex in the Forbidden Zone.* Unwin Hyman Paperbacks, London.
20. Dale, P. (1993) BAC Booklet *Guidelines for Counsellors: Counselling Adults who were Abused as Children.*

Disabilities and Chronic Illnesses

In 1973 the National Fund for Research into Crippling Diseases established a committee on the sexual relationship problems of people with disabilities. It was given the acronym 'SPOD'. A survey commissioned by SPOD in 1975 investigated a sample of 212 people with disability living in Coventry. The survey found that 54% of these people with disability said they were currently experiencing difficulties in their sexual lives. A further 18% had done so since the onset of their disability and had either overcome the problem or come to terms with it. In about 45% the sexual problem was attributed to physical factors; in 15% to predominantly psychological factors and 30% to a combination of the two.

Physical conditions which affect sexuality can be divided into two main groups (Hamilton, 1978)

1. Those in which sexual function is potentially normal but the expression of it may be made difficult by physical discomfort, pain, muscle spasm and involuntary movement. this group includes chronic illness such as arthritis, heart and lung disease, cerebral palsy, muscular dystrophy.

2. Those in which abnormal sexual function is caused by the illness itself, drugs given or by operations performed to treat the illness.

This group includes spinal cord damage, spina bifida, diabetes and operations to remove cancer of the bowel. In these conditions the ability of the man to have or maintain an erection can be lost and the normal sequence of ejaculation and accompanying orgasm may not take place. Mental conditions such as depression also come into this category.

Psychological effects of disability and chronic illness are of enormous importance in relationships and in sexual development and expression.

Someone who has a disability or illness whether visible or invisible may suffer from embarrassment, loss of self esteem and self worth, self disgust and feeling sexually unattractive with a poor body image.

Other people may react badly to a disability so damaging relationships. When this happens in childhood sexual development will be adversely affected. When the disability arises in adulthood existing relationships may be seriously affected. A sexual relationship may change to one which is more child-parent, or nurse-patient rather than adult-adult. In counselling a couple may be helped to regain a belief in the adulthood of the disabled or ill partner.

Loss of any function gives rise to grief for the damaged individual and for the partner. These losses, may include loss or damage to sexual functioning, loss of the healthy body and loss of the previous relationship. Grief for the losses has to be worked through before new ways of living can be successful. Counselling may have a crucial role to play in facilitating grieving.

It is only after the mourning process has taken place that new forms of sexual activity can be satisfactory.

The existence of a life threatening illness such as cancer can disrupt the sexual relationship with the healthy partner feeling guilty about seeking sexual pleasure in such circumstances.

There are people whose sexual function is normal but whose body image has been damaged in some way by illness, operation or accident so as to make them feel disfigured and sexually unattractive. Included in this group are women who have had a breast removed (mastectomy) for breast cancer. Not only do they have to contend with the disability and anxiety associated with the disease (including the treatment) but also with the feelings of losing whatever the breast signified for them: femininity, warmth, motherhood, or love perhaps, depending on the individual. A loss of confidence and depression may follow. Chronic skin diseases such as eczema and psoriasis (though not life threatening) can also be a source of much sexual unhappiness for similar reasons. Some operations as already mentioned damage sexual functions by destroying nerve fibres. Included here is prostatectomy in the man. The degree of damage is determined by the type of operation performed. Erectile problems are more common when the prostate is removed through the abdomen. In all types of operation however there are difficulties with ejaculation resulting in 'retrograde ejaculation', that is, ejaculation into the bladder. Pre- and post-operative counselling is needed.

Adults who have been born damaged or disfigured in some way may have suffered more from parental and social rejection than from the deformity or physical condition itself. They may also have suffered many years of surgical procedures which affect their body image and belief in their own attractiveness. Also there may be a sense that their bodies do not belong to them but are somehow public property to be disposed of by others.

Some Common Medical Conditions

Heart Attacks

There can be anxiety about the effects of sexual activity on the medical condition felt by both the person affected and the partner. There is a fear that sexual excitement will lead to another attack. Such issues have to be discussed with a knowledgeable doctor but this may not be easy for either of the partners involved. After a heart attack provided that sexual activity is taken gently and avoided after a substantial meal, no harm should occur. Drugs such a coronary dilators can be used before intercourse and if pain occurs then sexual activity should stop. The couple my need to change the way they make love, for instance, with the woman taking a more active role if her partner has had a heart attack. This has to be discussed carefully with both parties.

Diabetes

This illness is becoming increasingly common. It is feared by men as a cause of impotence. It only causes impotence when there is vascular and neurological damage in severe diabetes. However, the psychological effects of the condition being diagnosed are often profound. Thus impotency may occur only after the actual diagnosis is made. Counselling for both partners in this situation is required to explore what diabetes means to them and what their fears are about it.

Impotence occasionally may be the presenting symptom in some cases of diabetes. The majority of studies carried out on women with diabetes have shown little impairment of sexual function though they are more prone to vaginal infections when their diabetes is not well controlled.

Multiple Sclerosis

In this illness the nerve fibres anywhere in the nervous system can lose their outer covering (myelin). The effects are quite unpredictable and vary in different individuals. It might be quite localised and has a tendency to come and go leading to remissions and relapses. The outlook is extremely uncertain.

Sexual problems are common but not universal. They can result from non-specific consequences of the illness: tiredness, weakness, fatigue, depression, muscle spasm, pain. Feelings about loss of control can be important. There can be specific effects on the desire or sexual function of nerve damage. Impotence can present in different forms, for example erection in response to fantasies can be lost whilst erection in response to genital touching be maintained. Ejaculation can be impaired in the presence of normal erections.

Epilepsy

Lack of sexual interest and desire is the most commonly reported problem in people with epilepsy. There is also evidence that women have difficulty in responding to sexual stimulation and men have problems establishing normal erections. It is uncertain how far these difficulties have to do with epilepsy itself or with the effects of anti-convulsant drugs. Epilepsy carries considerable social stigma and children with epilepsy are likely to be over-protected. They may lack self confidence and fear rejection or fear the effects of sexual excitement because of its similarity to epileptic phenomena.

Drugs and Sexual Function

Some drugs used for therapeutic purposes can affect sexual function. For example, drugs used to treat high blood pressure can cause a variety of sexual difficulties in men ranging from erectile problems to delay in ejaculation and loss of interest in sex. Major tranquilisers and antidepressants including Prozac can reduce sexual desire in both sexes, whilst the tranquilisers can inhibit ejaculation in men. Anticonvulsants (apart from carbamazapine) decrease sexual desire. The oral contraceptive pill affects sexual interest in a minority of women making them less interested. The majority of women, however, show no or minimal effects with the pill. It is uncertain how the pill affects sexual interest. It is thought it may have to do with altering the woman's mood. (for further detailed information on sexuality and illness see Bancroft J, 'Human Sexuality and its Problems'. Churchill Livingstone, 2nd edition 1989 and Julia Segal: Counselling People with Disabilities/Chronic Illnesses in : Handbook of Counselling in Britain. Eds Windy Dryden, Ray Wolfe and David Charles-Edwards pp 329-346 Tavistock/Routledge London (1989))

Learning Disability

Approximately 3% of the population have learning difficulty or mental handicap. The majority of children with learning difficulties have parents who are within the average range of intelligence. The main causes of mental handicap are brain damage and Down's Syndrome.

People with metal handicap but unaffected by physical difficulties do not usually have any problems with sexual functioning apart from those caused by ignorance, fear and the effects of their upbringing. It is unfortunate that certain myths have been used to prevent the giving of information about sex and more generally, discussion of relationships of all kinds particularly where loss is concerned. These myths include:

*   people with mental handicap have no sexual desires;
*   they are 'sex maniacs' and have insatiable desires;
*   they are sexually deviant;
*   they are incapable of dealing with sex responsibly;
*   their children would be born damaged physically or mentally so they should not have them;
*   they are overgrown children and should be treated as such;
*   they don't have feelings like we do.

Ignoring the sexuality of those with learning disability can lead to behaviour such as exposure of genitals or masturbating in public places, which may bring the person unnecessary and painful contact with the law. This only reinforces the view that those with mental handicap are deviant. Increasing recognition has been given to the fact that sexual abuse of people with learning disability is fairly common which can worsen their mental condition (Brown and Craft, 1989 and Sinasson, 1992)

Issues for the client

*   The client may incorporate the views of society and feel their condition means they have no right to a sexual life.
*   The client may have different realistic and unrealistic beliefs about the condition which may contribute to difficulties in relationships. If intercourse is impossible, for example the client may feel s/he has no other way to express sexual feelings.

- The reaction of professionals (from past negative experiences) may be feared by the client.
- A client rejected in infancy as a result of some physical or mental condition may fear closeness as a prelude to rejection and create rejection in order to obtain a sense of mastery over the painful experiences.
- Past griefs and losses may not have been mourned as a result of unrealistic social expectations towards people with disabilities, mental or physical. This can affect emotional relationships. People with learning difficulties are often excluded from participation in discussion of painful emotions in particular grief and loss by their families and other care givers. This can seriously affect their beliefs about themselves, their bodies, their sexuality and their mental condition.

Issues for the Counsellor

- There is a need for affirmation of the right of every person, whatever their physical or mental condition, to sexual life.

  The counsellor needs to believe that it is possible that someone could love and care for the client however they look or behave. Difficulties believing this may need to be taken up with the client as well as the supervisor.
- The counsellor needs to accept that sex does not just mean sexual intercourse.
- Permission may need to be given by the counsellor for what is possible and exploring other ways of making love.
- The role of sexual fantasy should be explored by both counsellor and client. This requires sensitivity as people are often more embarrassed discussing their fantasies than what they actively do sexually.
- Specialist advice may be needed, e.g. for medical treatments, the use of sex aids, vibrators, contraceptive and genetic counselling.

  The counsellor could attend a course run by SPOD or the Family Planning Association. The latter runs courses for those involved in the care of those with learning disability.
- The counsellor may need to grieve alongside the client for past suffering which was never acknowledged. This may include grief for the losses the client believes their birth caused their parents.

Parents of Children with Disabilities

Having a child with a disability or chronic illness can affect the relationship between the parents. Sexual problems are common resulting from a number of factors. There is the physical and mental strain of looking after an ill or disabled child. There can be guilt about having such a child and feelings that sex, the womb or the relationship is damaging. There may be a denial of sexual feelings and pleasure as a form of self-punishment since these resulted in a damaged child. Rejecting and unloving feelings towards the child hidden or acknowledged, may cause difficulties in the parent's relationship. The wish to protect the child (and the self) from these damaging feelings may result in overcompensation so that the child is smothered and overprotected. This may lead to great difficulty in allowing the child to grow up and separate from them. A 'martyr complex' may develop with the parents sacrificing their own interests and those of other children to the damaged child. Siblings may resent the attention shown to the child.

Case History 1

Mr and Mrs I were referred to a psychosexual clinic by their general practitioner for 'sexual difficulties'. It appeared that both of them were avoiding sex though claiming that they were interested in it. They had two children, a daughter of 14 and a boy of 12 with Down's Syndrome. Mrs I was anxious about him and always kept their bedroom door open 'in case he got ill in the night'. Shutting the bedroom door to allow themselves to have privacy appeared too difficult. At first it seemed that both of them agreed to this situation. At a subsequent session Mr I revealed that the school which their son attended had suggested that it would be good for him to go away on holiday with a school party. Mrs I could not let him go 'something might happen'. Mr I got angry about this an argument ensued with Mrs I bursting into tears saying 'no one understood'. Eventually Mrs I was able to say that it was Mr I persuading her to have sex without using contraception (telling her he would be careful) that had resulted in the conception of their son. She had enjoyed that sexual occasion but after their son was born she blamed herself and her sexual enjoyment. She could not respond to her husband's sexual advances and he developed premature ejaculation. Sex took place less and less often.

Sharing their grief about their son which they had not done properly before, acknowledging that he was more capable than he was given credit for and that they had both rejected their daughter, enabled them to shut the bedroom door and let their son have more independence.

Case History 2

Mrs J was referred by her general practitioner to a psychosexual clinic with a loss of interest in sex which he thought was the result of taking the pill. She cried almost continually during the first session. In between sobs she talked about her son who had cystic fibrosis. It was her responsibility to give him physiotherapy twice a day. Her husband, she said, was a good man but he never helped her with their son. In fact, he acted as though he did not exist. Mr J was invited to attend the next session. It took several meetings to get through the wall of denial about his son's condition and the effect it had on him. The change began in their relationship when he broke down and wept for the son he actually had and the son he had hoped to have. They were both then able to share their grief and comfort each other. Mr J began to help Mrs J. Her resentment of him disappeared and she was able to show her love sexually.

References

1. Hamilton, A (1978) *The sexual Problems of the Disabled* British Journal of Family Planning 4(1)

2. Bancroft, J. (1989) *Human Sexuality and its Problems* Churchill Livingstone. 2nd Edition.

3. Segal, J. (1989) *Counselling People with Disabilities/Chronic Illnesses* in: Handbook of Counselling in Britain. (eds) Windy Dryden, Ray Woolfe and David Charles-Edwards pp. 329-346. Tavistock/Routledge, London

4. Brown, H and Craft, A. (1989) *Thinking the Unthinkable.* FPA Education Unit.

5. Sinasson, V. (1992) *Mental Handicaps and the Human Condition: New Approaches from the Tavistock.* Free Association Books, London.

Homosexuality

Profound changes in social attitudes towards homosexuality have taken place in the last 20 years. Homosexual relationships and practices are increasingly being accepted as another form of sexual behaviour rather than as abnormal, and more importantly, perhaps, as 'another form of human living and loving'. This change is largely due to the Gay Liberation Movement though individual homosexuals had worked courageously before the Movement had established itself in order to get the law changed in this country. Prior to the 1967 Sexual Offences Act which legalised sexual activity between two consenting males over 21, homosexuals went in fear of blackmail and homosexuality was seen as an illness to be treated if not a sin to be punished. In 1974 the American Psychiatric Association decided that homosexuality should no longer be regarded as a psychiatric illness. In 1993 the age of consent was lowered to 18.

The greater tolerance that had begun to be shown towards homosexuals is now in danger of being lost through the advent of Acquired Immune Deficiency Syndrome (AIDS) which in Western countries initially affected mainly homosexuals. Further ammunition has been provided for those who are anti-homosexual. The gay community itself bewildered, shocked and frightened, has nevertheless responded quickly in a responsible and caring way, alerting the wider public to the changes and advocating a change in sexual behaviour among homosexuals to minimise the risk of contracting the disease.

Causes

Homosexuals themselves are understandably irritated that so much attention is given to trying to find the 'causes' of homosexuality, seeing this as a reflection of society's anxiety about it. However not to do so may preclude rational discussion and also exacerbate prejudices by allowing myths to prevail. There is no evidence of physical differences nor of endocrine or hormonal difference so that homosexuals cannot be distinguished physically despite popular views to the contrary. In 1993 scientists claimed to have found a genetic basis for homosexuality though there is no gay gene.

Freud suggested a theory of constitutional bi-sexuality, that is an innate predisposition to the same-sex or opposite-sex partners. The choice between the two, he considered was determined by experiential factors in childhood. Later psychoanalysts (Bieber, 1962; Socarides, 1968) have emphasised the experiential factors. According to their view, there is unconscious guilt and anxiety related to heterosexuality which may force an individual to become homosexual. This guilt and anxiety are caused by a seductive, over-protective mother and father who is weak, hostile or absent from home. Analysts however, are likely to be treating only those homosexuals who, for whatever reason, are distressed by their homosexuality. The fact that many heterosexuals share a similar family pattern and a close mother-child relationship would seem to argue against these theories. Other authors (Bell and Weinburg, 1978) have stated 'homosexual adults who have come to terms with their homosexuality, who do not regret their sexual orientation and who can function effectively and socially, are no more distressed psychologically than are heterosexual men and women.'

Why has Western society been so exercised about homosexuality? Religious influences – where the emphasis on 'natural' sex and condemnation of all forms of non-reproductive sex – have obviously been the most significant. More subtle influences can be traced to the fear of homosexual feelings in oneself. There has also been a confusion between homosexuality and paedophilia; while some homosexuals may show a preference for children – as indeed do some heterosexuals – the majority do not.

Issues for the Client

*   The client may be uncertain as to whether the counsellor will be homophobic and whether he or she will give unbiased help.
*   The client may experience problems to do with self-acceptance and acceptance of homosexuality as a viable way of life.
*   There may be a sexual dysfunction with a current relationship.
*   The client may wish to change sexual orientation. Fewer homosexuals are presenting for treatment for this. It may be that the client has incorporated society's negative view and feels that homosexuality is not compatible with a loving relationship.
*   The client may have an understandable fear of AIDS.
*   The client may have mixed feelings towards heterosexuals, heterosexuality and its social dominance.

Issues for the Counsellor

- Counsellors should try to be aware of what their own attitudes and feelings are regarding homosexuality. Tolerance is not acceptance. (Ways of examining attitudes might be to contact a local gay group or invite a speaker or arrange role-play sessions.) If the counsellor is not happy to see a homosexual client, referral to a homosexual organisation is advisable.

- The counsellor needs to accept that homosexuals are people first with need and feelings. The counsellor should be aware that they may present with problems which have nothing to do with their sexual orientation such as involvement in an unhappy relationship, a loved one may leave or die. There may be difficulty in making relationships.

- There may be a sexual dysfunction, e.g. problems with sustaining an erection which requires sex therapy.

- The counsellor may be faced with a client who wishes to change their orientation. There will need to be a careful exploration of the possible reasons for this. If these are to do mainly with the incorporation of society's negative attitudes, the counsellor can allow an opportunity for the client's homosexuality to be looked at positively.

  The client who persists with the request needs to be told that the possibility of this depends very much on the degree of heterosexual interest and attraction.

  Behaviour therapy for this consists of attempts to enable a relationship with the opposite sex using a fantasy approach (encouraging heterosexual fantasies with masturbation) desensitisation approach (if for instance a man has a phobia of female genitals) and help with social skills. If a male client has a female partner she can be involved in couple therapy and instructed in a behavioral programme similar to that of heterosexual dysfunctional couples. Referral to a psychology department specialising in such treatment will be needed.

  Psychoanalysis over a period of many years may result in a real lasting change in sexual orientation from homosexual to heterosexual but for most people, a) this is not a viable option and b) this outcome is not guaranteed.

- The partner who discovers that their partner is homosexual may need help. Individuals who have strong homosexual and fairly strong heterosexual feelings can be faced with confusion and conflict as illustrated in one of the cases presented below.

Case Histories

Possible denial of homosexuality

Mrs F was 27 years old and had been married for two years. She presented at a family planning clinic with non-consummation. Her husband was a 40 year old clergyman. They had had a romantic courtship and shared many intellectual interests. She was helped to examine her vagina and stretch her hymen and many of her fears and anxieties were overcome. However the marriage was not consummated due to her husband's impotence. Her husband anxiously phoned the therapist on one occasion to say he was not impotent as he was having an affair with another woman – it was his wife's problem. Meeting the husband revealed that he was extremely anxious. He tried to hide his anxiety by being aggressive and manipulative. he attacked the professional integrity of the therapist. He came from an intensely religious family that seemed to be without much warmth or intimacy. He felt his father was contemptuous of his mother. It became evident that his heterosexual experience (apart from that with his wife) was practically non-existent. The slight (according to him) homosexual experience at boarding school was overlaid with such guilt and abhorrence that he refused to discuss it.

The marriage was annulled at the husband's request on the grounds of non-consummation. The therapist felt that there was a strong possibility that the husband was homosexual but because of the enormous anxiety surrounding this, it was not possible to explore this and it was considered better not to do so.

Problem of Self-Acceptance

Mr G was a young man from a deeply religious background. He presented himself at a clinic saying he wished to change sex since he did not feel attracted to girls. He was extremely shy and spoke so softly it was sometimes difficult to hear him. It took many sessions before enough trust and confidence could be built up between Mr G and the counsellor so that he could talk of his homosexual experiences and even longer for him to admit his own sexual attraction to other men. During this time he tried to make a relationship with a girl and was able to have intercourse with her very occasionally but got no joy from it; nor could he ejaculate. He eventually ended the relationship. He knew he could never share his true feelings with his family. They would, he felt, reject and disown him. His sexual feelings also brought him into conflict with his religious beliefs. Eventually he was referred at his own request to a homosexual counsellor. After several years Mr G has become a more self-assured and confident young man. He accepted sadly that he had to lead a double life where his family was concerned but he felt his present situation was preferable to the one he experienced when he first came to the counsellor.

Conflict of Feelings

Mr H came with a dilemma. He knew himself to be a homosexual and had had an intensive love affair with another man at college which ended when his family found out. All hell was let loose and various relatives took him to one side, telling him it was 'just a phase'. He formed a relationship with a girl of whom he was very fond. They had intercourse regularly which he quite enjoyed, but it did not have the passionate intensity and sense of fulfilment that occurred with his homosexual lover. His dilemma was that he very much wanted to marry and have children but felt he could not share his homosexual feelings with his girlfriend. The dilemma remained unsolved.

Lesbianism

While male homosexuality has been written about and investigated extensively not so much attention has been paid to lesbianism (female homosexuality) until very recent years. The picture is perhaps confused by some feminists consciously choosing to become lesbians (political lesbians) as a way of making a statement about men, that is that they do not need them and they do not wish to have any sexual relationship with them. However, it is unclear whether such lesbian women feel no sexual attraction towards men. It is also becoming evident that some lesbians have become disenchanted with such relationships, finding that issues of power, dominance/submission, and possessiveness are as much a feature of a female sexual relationship as they are of male/female relationships (Defries, 1978). Clients in violent or abusive relationships may need considerable help to handle their disillusionment and the discovery of their own violence and abusiveness if previously they attributed this solely to men.

Causes

As with male homosexuality the exact causes of lesbianism are not known. Many girls go through a lesbian phase – having crushes on older women, the idealized person they would like to be. Lesbian women have not been shown to be different to heterosexual women in terms of genetics, anatomy or hormones. Psychoanalytical observation has offered some patterns and tentative explanations of lesbianism. As with male homosexuals it has to be remembered that these theories derive from the analytical work with distressed lesbian women who seek help. The picture portrayed by such women of their parents shows a brutal insensitive father, an idealised yet controlling mother and a denial of any loving or complementariness between parents. The woman unconsciously identifies with her father and seeks an idealised woman partner (for further exploration of this see McDougall in Rosen, 1979).

Lesbian women rarely present themselves for help at psychosexual clinics, perhaps for the same reasons as homosexual men, fearing prejudice. They also rarely present to change their orientation.

Issues for the Counsellor

* As with male homosexuality the counsellor will need to look at their own attitudes, assumption and prejudices.

For example, it is often assumed that children growing up in a lesbian household will be damaged psychologically. An interesting study (Golumbok et al., 1983) explored some of the issues relating to this. 27 lesbian women with children were compared with 27 single heterosexual women with children. The women and children were interviewed as well as teachers of the children.

The two groups did not differ in terms of their gender identity, sex role behaviour or sexual orientation. Also they did not differ on most measures of emotions, behaviour and relationships.

The authors admit though that nearly all the children had been born into a heterosexual household and most has spent at least two years there. Interestingly the children from lesbian households had more contact with their fathers than did those from single parent households. Only a few women were definitely negative in their attitude towards men. It might be postulated that a child raised in a man-hating world, whether lesbian or heterosexual, would have damaged relationships with men and with the masculine part of the self.

* Counsellors need to recognise that not all women who explore lesbian feelings will develop a lesbian identity.

* Counsellors need to remember that women will experience problems which are not related to the fact that they are lesbian and for which they may need help, such as the loss or death of a loved one, financial and employment problems.

- There may be a sexual problem, e.g. difficulty in having an orgasm for which Masters and Johnson techniques can be helpful.

- As with all relationships (hetero- or homosexual) there may be an over-investment in 'sameness'. Difference rather than being celebrated is feared and seen as rejection. This happens when individuals feel insecure and lack self-esteem and self-worth.

References

1. Bieber, I (1962) *Homosexuality: A Psychoanalytical Study of Male Homosexuals.* New York: Basic Books.
2. Socarides, CW (1968) *The Overt Homosexual.* New York: Grune & Stratton.
3. Bell, A & Weinberg, M (1978) *Homosexuality: A Study of Diversity Among Men & Women.* New York: Simon & Schuster.
4. Bancroft, J. (1989) *Human sexuality and its Problems.* Churchill Livingstone, 2nd ed.
5. Defries, Z (Jan. 1978) *Political Lesbianism & Sexual Politics.* Journal of the American Academy of Psychoanalysis, 6(1), 71-78.
6. McDougall, J. (1979) *The Homosexual Dilemma: A Clinical & Theoretical Study of Female Sexuality* in 'Sexual Deviation', ed. Rosen, I. 2nd ed. Oxford University Press.
7. Golumbok, S, Spencer, A & Rutter, M. (1983) *Children in lesbian and single parent households.* Psychosexual & Psychiatric Appraisal. Journal of Child Psychology & Psychiatry, 24(4), 507-572.

Sexual Minorities

What has been regarded as normal and therefore acceptable sexual behaviour has varied widely among different cultures and at different times. In Western society, under Judaeo-Christian influence, it has been customary to regard any form of sexual behaviour other than straightforward heterosexual genital intercourse as deviant or perverted and in some cases unlawful. The importance of reproductive sex was stressed: 'be fruitful and multiply'; thus oral sex, anal intercourse, masturbation and homosexuality have been regarded as perversions since they did not lead to the creation of a life. As such they were put alongside rape, paedophilia and bestiality.

Chesser (1971) suggested a new dividing line in sexual behaviour between those acts where both partners consent (social) and those perpetrated against another's will (anti-social). The former would include sexual intercourse, mutual masturbation, oral sex, homosexuality, flagellation, fetishism, transvestism (cross-dressing) and anal intercourse: the latter would include exhibitionism, voyeurism, indecent assault, rape and offences against children. All acts in the anti-social group are also sexual offences as they involve exploitation and possible violence to another person. These will be looked at separately.

Apart from oral sex, mutual masturbation and female homosexuality, all other sexual behaviours are carried out by men. The reasons for this are unknown but possibly relate to the anxiety which surrounds potency and the ability to sustain an erection. Having an erection is not a willed process under conscious control.

The sexual behaviours to be discussed in this section are those relating to sadomasochism (flagellation), fetishism and transvestism. Before looking at each in turn certain characteristics need to be mentioned.

1. These sexual behaviours are manifested in varying degrees of intensity. Their frequency is often related to the stress experience in other areas of life, e.g. marital difficulties or job pressure.

2. There is an overlap in the various behaviours. Thus there can be a fetishistic aspect to cross dressing with certain kinds of garments being selected.

3.   The behaviours or acts are compulsive, ritualistic and repetitive. The performance of them appears to provide psychological relief. If a man is prevented from carrying out these acts he can become severely depressed.

4.   They tend to be associated with much fantasising and sexual day dreaming of a bizarre nature.

5.   The men who practice this behaviour tend to feel sexually unattractive, inferior and avoid sexual competition. This is far from the popular view that they are sexually very potent and filled with insatiable desire. In fact such men, believing themselves undesirable, can have difficulty in making or sustaining sexual and loving relationships. Hence there is a great reliance on prostitutes.

6.   The men are usually heterosexual, married with children. However sexual intercourse of itself is not as exciting and fulfilling as the other behaviours. This puts great stress on the partner.

7.   The men themselves rarely present for treatment at psychosexual clinics. They do not consider they have a problem. It is usually the partner who seeks help when some breaking point has been reached. She may have hoped that the behaviour would have lessened with time. As the years go by and the behaviour continues or increases with frequency, her tolerance can be exceeded. He may insist that she be more involved, with her sexual needs ignored unless she agrees.

8.   It may be extremely difficult for the man to change his behaviour unless he is motivated to do so.

Causes of these behaviours

What causes these behaviours is unknown for certain. Various theories have been put forward from psychoanalytic work with men who have presented themselves for treatment. A broad outline is offered here; for more detailed accounts readers are referred to Rosen, 1979, Storr, 1957, Klein, 1985. Psychoanalysis regards such behaviours as perversions.

1.   The mothers of these men are experienced by them as loving but intrusive. They tend to idolise their sons and treat them as objects or as extensions of themselves.

2.   The fathers, though often present during the childhood of these men, were perceived by their sons as shadowy, ineffectual people.

3.   The masculine was denigrated in their homes. The men manifesting these behaviours Storr (1957) contends, already feel castrated rather than fear it.

4.   These men display in the therapy a longing for fusion with the therapist but an intense fear of being annihilated related to the intrusiveness they experienced with their mothers. They do not develop a full sense of their own autonomy and have a fragile sense of self.

5.   The men are unconsciously fearful of their own aggression and its murderous quality. In order to cope with the destructive feelings towards their mothers in infancy and still preserve a relationship with her, their aggression was and continues to be converted into sadism. Thus the intention to destroy is converted into a wish to hurt and control. There is also sexualisation of the aggression. Glasser (see Rosen, 1979) believes that psychic disintegration will occur if the behaviours are not carried out since the behaviour forms an integral part of the personality and is not an isolated phenomena. Hence his view that sex serves as a servant to the psyche in these situations. This has important therapeutic implications for both the man and his partner. The partner may have convinced herself that it is only the behaviour that needs changing and may find difficulty accepting that this is not and cannot be an easy or straightforward process.

6.   The problems have their origins in early infant life. This may explain why these behaviours are difficult to change.

Treatment

If the man is willing to attend, the couple can be seen together to try to effect some meaningful compromise of his behaviour (its frequency; its degree).

Their sexual relationships need to be strengthened – modified Masters and Johnson techniques focusing on sensual pleasuring can be tried.

Assertion training for the man can be tried to enable him to feel more effective as a man.

If the man will attend he could be encouraged to seek psychotherapy though this treatment will be a long process.

Where the woman attends alone and the man refuses to attend, she will need help to understand her involvement in the relationship. Often these women have not felt secure about their sexuality and have chosen their partner because he felt sexually safe and kind. They may need help to leave the relationship.

Sadomasochism

Sexual pleasure is derived from the infliction of pain (sadism) or the reception of pain (masochism). Hardcore pornography consists largely of sadomasochistic acts. (The brutal sadist who may commit murder will obviously be included under sexual offences)

Within marriage degrees of sadomasochism seem to be tolerated. Thus if a man's potency depends on or is enhanced by sadomasochistic fantasies, his wife may be willing to participate, for example, in bondage where the partner is tied up and submits to sexual stimulation. Problems arise when the behaviour becomes more extreme with the man wanting to beat the woman to inflict injury or wants her to do the same.

Some men with masochistic needs indulge in practices which are life-threatening, such as partial self-strangulation.

The Kleinan view 1985) of sadomasochism sees it as related to split off parental figures to which the self relates. Thus it may feel like the self is watching the father or mother (in the self) being punished by the sadomasochistic act. The sadomasochistic act can be seen as an enactment of a very cruel and frightening view of sexual intercourse either between the parents or between the self and another much more powerful person.

Fetishism

Erotic arousal is centred on an object or part of the body or an article of clothing. The fetish is used as a talisman to ensure an erection. There are degrees of fetishism from the mild fairly common condition in which the fetish ensures potency to the extreme form where the fetish replaces the partner and is used for masturbation. The fetish is usually quite specific and linked to someone closely involved with the man in his childhood and is constant over time, e.g. rubber pants, corsets, high heeled shoes. Some fetishes are associated with sadomasochistic practices such as being trodden on by leather boots. the man may keep his fetish a secret and merely fantasises on the object. Problems may arise when he asks his partner to participate in his fantasies such as dressing up in special clothing. Wives may not mind this within limits but if he insists that she wears clothes which make her look or feel ridiculous all the time she may seek help. She may also seek help where the fetish becomes such an obsession that her husband withdraws from any sexual contact with her. Winnicott (1953) equated the fetish with the 'transitional object' used in childhood to cope with separation from mother. However, Greenacre (1979) disagrees and sees the fetish compensating for an illusion of some actual impairment of the genitals.

Case History

A married woman in her 30s attended a psychosexual clinic. In between tears she talked of her husbands obsession with corsets. He had all the corset magazines sent to him and insisted that she wear tight corsets. He would then come up surreptitiously behind her and slip his hand under her buttocks and pull on the corsets. he would then either masturbate or have intercourse. He had never had intercourse in marriage without this preliminary. They had been married nine years and did not have children. She had been a fat unattractive teenager and her husband was her first boyfriend. In order to appear slimmer she wore corsets. One of the reasons she married her husband was that he found her attractive despite her obesity. Reassured about this she began to slim and not wear corsets. The husband's sympathetic manner changed and he would verbally abuse and insult her. He insisted she wear corsets and restrictive clothing. She felt ridiculous and used. As she lost weight men in her office found her attractive. Having lost the feeling that her husband loved her, she felt she could no longer comply with his wishes. This led to more and more arguments until she finally left him. The husband's history (as given by the wife) was of a lonely childhood, rejected by his parents and sent to boarding schools where some women teachers made a fuss of him.

Transvestism: Cross Dressing

Some men get satisfaction in dressing up in women's clothing and in imitating women in various ways. If a man cannot act out his impulse he may become depressed. It is estimated that about 1-2% of the population are so affected. This inclination to dress up in women's clothes is laid down in early life. Some transvestites report that when they were young they were forced to dress in girl's clothes. The experiences were usually accompanied by feelings of fear and humiliation but also excitement. According to Storr (1957), the man assumes female dress not because he wishes to be a woman but because he wishes to obtain phallic power which is still felt to belong to the woman. Transvestisism tends to last throughout life beginning in childhood or after puberty. Changing into women's clothes is usually sexually stimulating and is accompanied by sexual fantasies and masturbation. It has a compulsive aspect to it and intense relief is experienced afterwards. For some transvestites merely dressing up as a woman and being accepted as one can give great satisfaction. Although a few may want to change sex, the majority seem happy to have two personae. Most transvestites are heterosexual and may be married with children. Some hide their transvestism from their wives; others tell their wives. The reaction of the women may vary – some are disgusted and want a divorce or will only agree to remain if the husband gives up his inclination; yet others will actively support their husbands in their cross dressing, buying clothes, wigs etc., for them. Transvestism often has the element of a fetish about it in that particular kinds of garments are selected.

The Beaumont Society exists to support and help transvestites and their families. It also provides opportunities for its members to cross dress in company.

Transsexualism : Problems of gender identity

Transsexualism refers to a disturbance of gender identity and difficulties with the assigned gender role. The person feels that their anatomy is incompatible with the psychological sexual identity. The condition seems to affect more men than women. The actual incidence is unknown but estimates of those seeking sex reassignment have ranged from 2 in 100,000 men and 1 in 400,000 women. In its extreme form the individual seeks help to change their gender identity by means of hormone treatment and surgery – the so-called sex change. The search for help can be a desperate one with the person going from doctor to doctor.

How transsexualism is caused is not known for certain. It is postulated for male transsexuals that as children they formed an intense close relationship with their mothers which excluded other members of the family. (Green, 1974, 1979). Yet other workers (e.g. Prince, 1978) have found that for the male transsexual the struggle to maintain a successful masculine identity is too great and there is the assumption that the change from male to female 'will reduce the disparity between expectation and performance'.

For a feminist perspective on transsexualism see Raymond (1979) who sees 'a society that produces sex-role stereotyping functions as the primary cause of transsexualism'. Surgery, as she notes, is only permitted when the person is able to pass as stereotypically 'masculine' or 'feminine'. Nevertheless the belief that changing from one sex to the other will improve their lot is very strong indeed for some people. Two types have been described (Stoller, 1979) primary where the male child from one year on behaves in a feminine manner and secondary where the man cross dresses initially then begins to experience the desire to be a woman.

Management of a person wishing to change sex

There are a few specialist centres in Britain and the United States that will perform sex change operations; about 2000 people have undergone them in the US.

Centres usually set conditions before they agree to operate, namely that the person must have lived as a member of the opposite sex for about two years and must have undergone hormonal treatment. This needs to be given for 1-2 years prior to the operation.

Surgery

For Male-to-Female Reassignment
The penis and testicles are removed. A vagina is fashioned using penile skin, the scrotal skin is used for forming the labia. Post operative complications are common and may be troublesome.

For Female-to-Male Transsexual
The surgical options are less satisfactory. Breasts, ovaries and womb are removed. the creation of penis and scrotum presents formidable difficulties.

Outcome of Sex Reassignment Surgery

Adequate long term follow-up studies of sex reassignment surgery are only recently appearing in the literature, Lundstrom et al. (1984) reviewed the follow-up literature. Among their conclusion were the following:

1.   an unsatisfactory result in 10-15% cases;

2.   approximately 5% of cases regret the surgery;

3.   female-to-male transsexuals fare better then male-to-female;

4. personal and social instability pre-operative is associated with unsatisfactory post-operative outcome;

5. the younger the age at which reassignment is requested, the better the outcome.

Female Perversions

Welldon (1988), a psychoanalyst, has challenged the view that the sexual perversions are only found in men. She considers that women demonstrate perverted behaviour through the whole body with self inflicted injuries as a relief from sexual anxiety. Anorexia and bulimia are other means used to attack the body. Motherhood can be used to exercise perverse attitudes towards offspring with the baby becoming a toy or thing to be abused, ravaged, discarded, cherished and idealised. Prostitution is seen as a perversion. Welldon contends that both prostitute and client become partners in minds and bodies in a vengeful and denigrating action against mother.

References

1. Chesser, E (1971) *The Human Aspects of Sexual Deviation.* London: Arrow Books.
2. Rosen, I (ed.) (1979) *Sexual deviation.* Oxford University Press: Oxford.
3. Khan, MMR (1979) *Alienation in Perversions.* Karnac Books, London.
4. Storr, A (1957) *The Psychology of Fetishism & Transvestism.* Journal of Analytical Psychology. Vol.2, No.2.
5. Klein, M. (1985) *Love, Guilt and Reparation.* The Hogarth Press, London. pp.210-218.
6. Glasser, M. (1979) *Some aspects of the role of aggression in the perversions* in 'Sexual Deviation'. Rosen (ed). Oxford University Press.
7. Glasser, M. (1993) *The Weak Spot in The Gender Conundrum.* Breen, D. (ed) Routledge; London.
8. Winnicott, D. (1953) *Transitional Objects Phenomena.* Int.J. Psycho-analysis, 34, 89.
9. Greenacre, P. (1979) *Fetishism in Sexual Deviation.* Rosen, I (ed.) Oxford University Press, Oxford.
10. Green, R. (1974) *Sexual Identity Conflict in Children and Adults.* Duckworth, London.
11. Green, R. (1979) *Childhood Cross-Gender Behaviour.* American Journal of Psychiatry 136: 106-108.
12. Prince, V. (1978) *Transsexuals and Pseudo-Transsexuals.* Archives of Sexual Behaviour 7: 263-272.
13. Raymond, J. (1979) *The Transsexual Empire.* Boston, MA: Beacon Press.
14. Stoller, R. (1979) *The Gender Disorders* in Rosen I (ed.) Sexual Deviation, Oxford University Press, Oxford.
15. Lundstrom, B et al. (1984) *Outcome of Sex Reassignment Surgery.* Acta Psychiatrica Scandinavica 70: 289-294.
16. Welldon, E. (1988) *Mother, Madonna, Whore.* London: Free Association Books.

Sexual Offences

The number of indictable sexual offences known to the police has increased over the last 30 years. In 1978 the number of indictable sexual offences was 22,367. In 1989 the number was 30,000. The commonest sexual offence was indecent assault on women (15,400). (Figures available from the Home Office).

Exhibitionism

This is the commonest of all sexual offences. There are over 3000 convictions per year. Most offenders are charged once. If they are charged a second time the outlook is poor. It is a male disorder. The genitals are exposed, usually to a girl or young woman and the reaction of horror and excitement induced gives the exhibitionist the satisfaction he seeks. He feels powerful for causing such a reaction. Exhibitionists are usually weak, insecure men. Unhappiness at home, stress and marital problems are often found to precipitate such behaviour. Some exhibitionists seem to have a compulsive need to get caught. These are the ones who exhibit themselves more than once in the same place. The element of danger involved in risking discovery may be a powerful sexual stimulant in itself.

Treatment

Both psychodynamic and behavioural methods (mainly aversion therapy) have been tried in the past with a measure of success. Nowadays the emphasis is on helping the individual build up or reinforce new and more adaptive behaviours rather than simply to eliminate the undesirable one (Bancroft, 1989) for example, social skills training, self-assertion training.

Rape

The number of cases notified to the police in 1989 was 3,305. 61% of rapes are by people known to the woman. 59% of rapes happen indoors. Women are often reluctant to report rape because of the ordeal of standing up in court and reliving a terrible experience and often being made to feel that they are to blame for its occurrence. Also, the police have not always been sympathetic to the women who report rape. Pressure from women's groups and rape crisis centres combined with the notoriety surrounding some cases has resulted in women police officers being delegated to interview the woman reporting the rape. Recognition is now being given to the fact that women can be raped by their husbands.

The Law and Rape

A man commits rape if:

a)   he has unlawful sexual intercourse with a woman without her consent by force, fear or fraud (Sexual Offences Act 1956) and

b)   at the time he knows she does not consent to intercourse or he is reckless as to whether she consents to it (Sexual Offences Act 1976).

The 1976 Act gave the right of anonymity to raped women (although at the discretion of the judge) and a direction that the woman's past sexual history should not be referred to unless the judge considers it relevant to the case.

Penetration of the vagina by hand or use of bottles and broom handles does not constitute rape; this would constitute grievous bodily harm. There are a number of myths about rape.

Myths

Nice girls don't get raped
Women enjoy rape
Rape is committed by maniacs
Women ask for rape 'They say no when they mean yes'
Women deserve rape
Women make false allegations of rape

Some Facts

1.   Women of all ages, races, social classes and life styles have been raped.

2.   Rape often involves beating and the use of sticks and knives.

3.   Women are raped in any situation, at home, out walking, at work. This contradicts the belief that rape occurs only late at night and that the woman deserves rape because she was running a risk.

4.   Of women confronted with a threat to their life or physical well-being, in one study 55% were submissive, 27% resisted, and 18% fought (Amir, 1971). This is important since the man may use a defence that the women consented. If she feared for her life she might well consent.

Women who have been raped, like the rest of society, believe it is their fault and wonder what they have done to provoke the attack and what they could have done to prevent or stop it. It is possible that the helplessness and impotence of being quite unable to control the situation feels even worse than the self-blame and guilt.

After a woman has been raped she may become agoraphobic and refuse to go out. She may lose her self-confidence. She can develop sexual difficulties and refuse sex with her partner since sexual intercourse recapitulates the attack. It may take months or even years to recover from the attack and some women never recover.

(When the first Rape Crisis Centre was opened in London in 1976, many of the women who contacted it had been raped many years before. The anger, pain and humiliation they felt was still very much in evidence.)

Helping the Raped – Issues for the Client

The women may initially either be in a state of shock or uncontrollably agitated or distressed. She may need others to take over the responsibilities of her day to day living.

The crisis precipitated by rape has similarities to that produced by bereavement or loss. Once the initial shock is passed the proper working through or mourning of the many losses involved is a crucial part of recovery. Earlier experience with a similar significance may be re-awakened by the event and may in turn need working through.

If a counsellor sees a woman soon after she has been raped she should be told not to clean herself or remove her clothes as this will remove the evidence (often the first thing, understandably, that the woman wants to do is to rid herself of the experience in the literal, physical sense.) The counsellor, if possible, should accompany the woman to the doctor and police station. The woman's physical state will be needed as evidence together with blood or semen – stained clothing. Sperm may not always be detected since some rapists fail to ejaculate. Examination shortly after rape will fail to reveal bruises since these may take hours to develop. Pregnancy tests and tests for sexually transmitted disease will need to be performed. Post-coital contraception can be given within 72 hours of the attack. Abortion may be necessary.

There are now several Rape Crisis centres to be found mainly in large cities. They have a telephone service and offer counselling and advice. They will also accompany the woman to the police to advise about legal help. The London Rape Crisis Centre has counselled 5,575 women and girls between the years 1972 and 1982 and taken a total of 6,472 calls.

After the shock may come denial, anger and self blame. The woman may give the appearance of having recovered and talk in a very detached way of the event, creating powerful feelings of horror and revulsion in the listener. Her fury may be directed both at the assailant and at others who failed to help or compounded her difficulties. She may go over and over in her mind ways she could have prevented the attack even if realistically this was not possible. She may lose her trust in the world, in men and in herself. She may feel spoiled and damaged with a loss of identity, particularly if she was abused as a child. She may lose her partner and other people's attitude to her may change as a result of their knowledge.

Issues for the Counsellor

- Counsellors need to be aware of the facts about rape and the harm that can be done physically and psychologically to the woman and her partner. Such clients need time and patience to tell what happened in their own way.

- The counsellor needs to affirm positively how the woman behaved at the time of the rape (how brave, how sensible, how she coped) and to challenge any assumptions that she provoked the attack. It needs to be made absolutely clear that there was no justification or excuse for the behaviour of the assailant. It can help to talk of her feelings of self blame as being a defence against her real helplessness and impotence in the face of the attack.

- When counselling women who have been raped, acknowledging the pain of it, giving sympathy, care and support especially if the counsellor is a woman is a relatively easy part of the task. The possibility of rape will have featured in most women's thoughts at some time either in relation to themselves or female relatives. However, without support, the counsellor may at times risk being overwhelmed by the material presented. Another aspect especially hard to cope with is the sense of being violated oneself. It is as if the woman relating the experience has to make the counsellor feel what she felt. This is not a conscious and deliberate action but an unconscious one. Nevertheless it can leave the counsellor feeling confused and hurt. For the client there is a strong and understandable wish for revenge and a wish to hurt the way she has been hurt, to regain a sense of power and control. The woman needs sustained support to regain her dignity and self-worth so as not to see herself simply as a victim.

- The client's partner and relatives may need help and support to deal with their feelings especially negative ones of blaming the woman. Again their feelings of blame can be a cover up for their own feelings of guilt and shame for not being able to prevent the attack and protect the victim.

- The counsellor needs to be aware of the long-term effects: sexual difficulties, depression and the bringing to the surface or pre-existing difficulties within the relationship/marriage.

- Where the rape was by the husband, the woman will need help to extricate herself from the marriage. The law has now recognised that a woman can be raped by her husband.

Paedophilia

Literally, paedophilia means the love of children. The man derives his erotic pleasures from contact with children either by exposing himself, touching their genitals and/or getting them to touch his or attempting penetration. The child, who can be male or female, is usually pre-puberty (6-11 years). Although the paedophile is portrayed as a dangerous sex maniac, in fact violence occurs in only a minority of cases. Studies show that the paedophile is much more likely to be known to the child (in some way) rather than be a complete stranger. The adult wants an emotional relationship with the child. When this fails the threat of physical force may be used.

Paedophiles have been divided into two groups (Burgess et al., 1978)

1. The fixated paedophile who has been primarily attracted to younger people from adolescence. Sexual relationships with adults tend to be avoided for fear of rejection and from feelings of inadequacy or inferiority. The offences are chronic and persistent. There are no feelings of guilt or shame and the sexual desires are experienced as compulsive.

2. The regressed paedophile originally preferred adult partners for sexual gratification. He often feels inadequate in the face of adult responsibilities and if the stress in his life is too great, for example, with his marriage or job he turns to a child for comfort. He is usually distressed and ashamed by his behaviour. Treatment is thus easier.

Treatment for the fixated paedophile is more difficult. He has been described as a psychological child in the physical guise of an adult with deep-seated feelings of inadequacy, poor impulse control and an inability to tolerate frustration.

It is possible that the child with whom the paedophile tries to make a relationship is in fantasy himself and the love he gives to the child is what he himself would have liked to receive. Offenders against children are typically heterosexual.

It has been recognised more recently that women too, can and do sexually abuse children.

Sexual Abuse

Sexual abuse is an enormous subject which has been widely written about (see *Counselling Adults who were Abused as Children* also in this series).

Issues for the Counsellor

It needs to be made clear to the woman (or man) that no child, no matter how apparently seductive, can be held responsible for sexual abuse occurring. This may be strongly resisted as it means confronting the child's belief in their own omnipotent power. This self blame, as in the case of rape, may seem preferable to facing the humiliation and impotence of the child's real helplessness in the face of the adult's demands.

References

1. Amir, M. (1971) *Patterns of Forcible Rape*. Chicago: University of Chicago Press.

2. Katz, S & Mazur, MA (1979) *Understanding Rape Victims: a synthesis of research findings*. New York: Wiley.

Useful Addresses

Institute of Psychosexual
Medicine 11 Chandos
Street Cavendish Square London
W1M 9DE 0171 580 0631
Provides lists of psychosexual
clinics run by National Health
Service.

British Association for Sexual and
Marital Therapists
PO Box 62
Sheffield S10 3TS
Provides lists of psychosexual
clinics and therapists (both NHS
and private) offering wide range of
treatment methods (SAE requested)

Relate
Herbert Gray College
Little Church Street
Rugby
Warwickshire CV21 3AP
01788 573241
Information of Marital Sexual
Therapy Clinics, for local branches
see Relate in local phone book.

Family Planning Association
Information Department
2-12 Pentonville Road
London N1 9FP
0171 837 5432

Beaumont Society
BM Box 3084
London WC1V 6XX
0171 730 7453
Support for Transvestites

Identity Counselling Service
Beauchamp Lodge
2 Warwick Crescent
Paddington
London W2 6NE
0171 289 6175
for those with identity problems
(gender dysphoria)

Sexual & Relationship
Problems of the Disabled (SPOD)
286 Camden Road
London N7 0BJ
0171 607 8851

Recommended Book List

Sexuality for Clients and Counsellors

Becoming Orgasmic: A sexual and personal growth programme for women. Julia Heiman and Joseph Lo Piccolo. Piatkus Books (1988)

*My Secret Garden:*Women's sexual fantasies. Nancy Friday. (1988) Quartet Books.

The Book of Love: Dr David Delvin, New English Library (1992) Revised Edition

The Joy of Sex: Alex Comfort. Quartet Books. (1975)

Massage and Loving: Anne Hooper. Unwin Hyman (1988)

Men and Sex: Bernie Zilbergeld. Fontana (1995)

Men in Love: Their secret fantasies. Nancy Friday. Arrow Books (1989)

Safer Sex: A new look at sexual pleasure. Peter Gordon and Louise Mitchell. Faber & Faber (1988)

Sex Problems: Your questions answered. Martin Cole and Windy Dryden. Macdonald Optime (1989)

Treat Yourself to Sex: A guide to good loving. Paul Brown and Carolyn Faulder. Penguin (1988)

Being Lesbian: Lorraine Trenchard. GMP Publishing (1989)

How to be a Happy Homosexual: Terry Sanderson. GMP Publishing (1989)

Living , Loving and Ageing: Wendy Greengross and Sally Greengross. Age Concern (1989)

Sexual Happiness for Men: Maurice Yaffe and Elizabeth Fenwick. Dorling Kindersley (1992)

Sexual Happiness for Women: Maurice Yaffe and Elizabeth Fenwick. Dorling Kindersley (1992)

Making the Most of Loving: Gill Cox and Sheila Dainow. Sheldon Press (1988)

Sex in Human Loving: Eric Berne, London. Andre Deutsch (1971)

Vaginismus Understanding and Overcoming the Block to Intercourse: Linda Valins. Ash Grove Press (1988)

Sexuality and Disability

Entitled to Love: Wendy Greengross. Melbray Press (1976)

Sexual Options for Paraplegics & Quadraplegics: Thomas Mooney. Little Brown & Co (1975)

Sexuality and Handicap: Ed.B.H.H. Dechesne, C.Pons and A.M.C.M. Schellen. Woodhead Faulkner (1985)

For the Counsellor

The Sexual Relationship: An Object Relations view of sex and the family: David E. Scharrf. Routledge, London (1982)

Object Relations Couple Therapy: David E. Scharrf and Jill Savege Scharff. Aronson, London (1991)

Human Sexuality & Its Problems: John Bancroft. Churchill Livingstone (1989) 2nd Edition

Introduction to Psychosexual Medicine: Ed. R.L.Skrine. Montana Press (1989)

Sex Therapy: A practical guide. Keith Hawton. Oxford University Press. (1988)

Sex Therapy in Britain: Martin Cole and Windy Dryden (eds). Open University Press (1988)

Sexuality & Birth Control in Community Work: Elphis Christopher. Tavistock 2nd Edition (1987)

Sex Directory: A guide to sexual problems and where to go for help. Compiled by Ann Darnborough and Derek Kinrade. Woodhead Faulkner (1988)

Insights into Troubled Sexuality: Prudence Tunnadine. Chapman and Hall (1992 Revised Edition.

Sex Education & Counselling for Mentally Handicapped People: Ann and Michael Craft (eds.) Costellos (1983)

Practice Issues in Sexuality & Learning Disabilities: Ed. Ann Craft (1994) Routledge

We Speak Ourselves: The experiences of gay men and women. Jack Bauscio. SPCK (1988)

Sexuality and its Discontents: Jeffrey Weeks. London. Routlege & Kegan Paul (1985)

[1] for further information on other studies, see Chapter 2 in Sex Therapy in Britain, edited by Martin Cole and Windy Dryden (1988)